Pressure Injuries Among Critical Care Patients

Editor

JENNY G. ALDERDEN

CRITICAL CARE NURSING CLINICS OF NORTH AMERICA

www.ccnursing.theclinics.com

Consulting Editor
CYNTHIA BAUTISTA

December 2020 • Volume 32 • Number 4

ELSEVIER

1600 John F. Kennedy Boulevard • Suite 1800 • Philadelphia, Pennsylvania, 19103-2899

http://www.theclinics.com

CRITICAL CARE NURSING CLINICS OF NORTH AMERICA Volume 32, Number 4
December 2020 ISSN 0899-5885, ISBN-13: 978-0-323-75707-2

Editor: Kerry Holland
Developmental Editor: Laura Fisher

Critical Care Nursing Clinics of North America (ISSN 0899-5885) is published quarterly by Elsevier Inc., 360 Park Avenue South, New York, NY 10010-1710. Months of issue are March, June, September, and December. Business and Editorial Offices: 1600 John F. Kennedy Blvd., Suite 1800, Philadelphia, PA 19103-2899. Periodicals postage paid at New York, NY and additional mailing offices. Subscription prices are $160.00 per year for US individuals, $428.00 per year for US institutions, $100.00 per year for US students and residents, $206.00 per year for Canadian individuals, $538.00 per year for Canadian institutions, $230.00 per year for international individuals, $538.00 per year for international institutions, $115.00 per year for international students/residents and $100.00 per year for Canadian students/residents. To receive student/resident rate, orders must be accompanied by name of affiliated institution, data of term, and the *signature* of program/residency coordinator on institution letterhead. Orders will be billed at individual rate until proof of status is received. Foreign air speed delivery is included in all *Clinics* subscription prices. All prices are subject to change without notice. **POSTMASTER:** Send address changes to *Critical Care Nursing Clinics of North America*, Elsevier Health Sciences Division, Subscription Customer Service, 3251 Riverport Lane, Maryland Heights, MO 63043. **Customer Service: 1-800-654-2452 (US and Canada); 314-447-8871 (outside US and Canada). Fax: 314-447-8029. E-mail:** JournalsCustomerService-usa@elsevier.com **(for print support) and** JournalsOnlineSupport-usa@elsevier.com **(for online support).**

Reprints. For copies of 100 or more of articles in this publication, please contact the Commercial Reprints Department, Elsevier Inc., 360 Park Avenue South, New York, New York, 10010-1710; Tel.: 212-633-3874, Fax: 212-633-3820, and E-mail: reprints@elsevier.com.

Critical Care Nursing Clinics of North America is covered in *MEDLINE/PubMed (Index Medicus), International Nursing Index, Nursing Citation Index, Cumulative Index to Nursing and Allied Health Literature,* and *RNdex Top 100.*

Contributors

CONSULTING EDITOR

CYNTHIA BAUTISTA, PhD, APRN, FNCS, FCNS
Associate Professor, Egan School of Nursing and Health Studies, Fairfield University, Fairfield, Connecticut, USA

EDITOR

JENNY G. ALDERDEN, PhD, APRN, CCRN, CCNS
Assistant Professor, University of Utah College of Nursing, Salt Lake City, Utah, USA

AUTHORS

JENNY G. ALDERDEN, PhD, APRN, CCRN, CCNS
Assistant Professor, University of Utah College of Nursing, Salt Lake City, Utah, USA

ELIZABETH A. AYELLO, PhD, MS, BSN, ETN, RN, CWON, MAPWCA, FAAN
Co-Editor-in-Chief, Advances in Skin & Wound Care, Philadelphia, Pennsylvania, USA; Executive Editor Emeritus, WCET® Journal, Perth Australia; Faculty, Faculty Emeritus, Excelsior College, School of Nursing, Albany, New York, USA; President, World Council of Enterostomal Therapists (WCET©) (Registered Charity UK); Senior Adviser, Hartford Institute for Geriatric Nursing, President, Ayello, Harris & Associates, Inc, New York, New York, USA

CHRISTINE T. BERKE, MSN, APRN-NP, CWOCN-AP
Nurse Practitioner, Center for Wound Healing and Ostomy Care, Nebraska Medicine, Omaha, Nebraska, USA

JOYCE M. BLACK, PhD, RN, FAAN
Professor, College of Nursing, University of Nebraska Medical Center, Omaha, Nebraska, USA

VIANNA BRODERICK, MD
Geriatrician, James A. Haley Veterans Hospital and Clinics, Tampa, Florida, USA

LINDA COWAN, PhD, APRN, FNP-BC, CWS
Associate Chief Nursing Service Research, Associate Director, VISN 8 Patient Safety Center of Inquiry, James A. Haley Veterans Hospital and Clinics, Tampa, Florida, USA

JILL COX, PhD, RN, APN-c, CWOCN
Clinical Associate Professor, Rutgers University School of Nursing, Newark, New Jersey, USA; Wound/Ostomy/Continence Advanced Practice Nurse, Englewood Health, Englewood, New Jersey, USA

BARBARA DELMORE, PhD, RN, CWCN, MAPWCA, IIWCC-NYU
Senior Nurse Scientist, Center for Innovations in the Advancement of Care (CIAC), Clinical Assistant Professor, Hansjörg Wyss, Department of Plastic Surgery, NYU Langone Health, New York, New York, USA

CARROLL GILLESPIE, MS, BSN, RN, CWOCN
Clinical Manager, Arjo, Inc, Addison, Illinois, USA

MARK GOETCHEUS, BSN, RN, CWON, CFCN, CDE
Program Manager, Wound, Ostomy, Limb Preservation, & Amputation Services, Harborview Medical Center, Seattle, Washington, USA

MELISSA L. HUTCHINSON, DNP, ARNP-CNS, CCNS, CWCN-AP, CCRN
Director, Wound Care Team, VA Puget Sound Healthcare System

NANCY MUNOZ, DCN, MHA, RDN, LD, FAND
Lecturer, UMass Amherst, Massachusetts, USA; Assistant Chief, Nutrition and Foodservice, VA Southern Nevada Healthcare System, North Las Vegas, Nevada, USA

ANN MARIE NIE, RN, MSN, APRN, FNP-BC, CWOCN
Board Member, National Pressure Injury Advisory Panel, Wound, Ostomy Care Team Nurse Practitioner, Children's Minnesota Hospital and Clinics, Minneapolis, Minnesota, USA

JOYCE PITTMAN, PhD, RN, ANP-BC, FNP-BC, CWOCN, FAAN
Associate Professor, College of Nursing, University of South Alabama, Mobile, Alabama, USA

ANDREA L. ROUFOGALIS, BSN, CWON
Wound Care Team, VA Puget Sound Healthcare System

FAYGAH SHIBILY, PhD, RN
Assistant Professor, Faculty of Nursing, King Abdulaziz University, Jeddah, Saudi Arabia

HOLLY VANCE, BSN, RN, CWON
Wound and Ostomy Clinical Nurse Educator, Harborview Medical Center, Seattle, Washington, USA

SUNNIVA ZARATKIEWICZ, PhD, RN, CWCN
Director, Professional Development and Nursing Excellence, Harborview Medical Center, Seattle, Washington, USA

Contents

> The first step in successful pressure injury (PI) prevention is the identification of appropriate risk factors. In the critically ill, determination of PI risk is multifactorial and clinically challenging, as there are many unique risk factors that confront this population. Empirically supported PI risk factors in the critical care population include age, diabetes, hypotension, compromised mobility, prolonged intensive care unit admission, mechanical ventilation and vasopressor administration. Future risk assessment using sophisticated data analytics combined with electronic medical information may result in earlier targeted PI prevention and will improve our understanding of risk factors that contribute to unavoidable PIs.

> Pressure injuries are areas of damage to the skin and underlying tissue caused by pressure or pressure in combination with shear. Pressure injury prevention in the critical care population necessitates risk assessment, selection of appropriate preventive interventions, and ongoing assessment to determine the adequacy of the preventive interventions. Best practices in preventive interventions among critical care patients, including skin and tissue assessment, skin care, repositioning, nutrition, support surfaces, and early mobilization, are described. Unique considerations in special populations including older adults and individuals with obesity are also addressed.

> Pressure injury treatments are tailored to the characteristics of the wound. Wound depth, exudate, presence of infection, and patient goals of care will guide appropriate dressing and treatment selection. The interprofessional team, patient, and family should collaborate to create a plan of care for wound healing.

> Pressure injury prevention in critically ill pediatric patients can be challenging. The current article discusses pressure injury prevention and treatment with attention to unique aspects of pediatric physiology that influence risk for pressure injury. Medical device–related pressure injuries

are particularly problematic in pediatric patients; therefore, this article presents best practice in preventing pediatric medical device-related pressure injuries. Treatment of pressure injuries is also discussed, with special attention to products that should be used with caution or avoided.

Medical device–related pressure injuries result from use of medical devices, equipment, furniture, and everyday objects in direct contact with skin and because of increased external mechanical load leading to soft tissue damage. The resultant pressure injury generally mirrors the pattern or shape of the device. The nurse and clinician must be hypervigilant of increased risk of pressure injuries with the use of these devices. This article provides evidence-based information regarding the most common devices that cause pressure injuries in adults and describes current best evidence-based prevention strategies. Evidence-based prevention strategies are key to minimizing the harm devices can cause.

Unstageable pressure injuries are widely understood to be full-thickness pressure injuries in which the base is obscured by slough and/or eschar. Correct identification of these pressure injuries can be challenging among health care professionals and, although treatments vary, débridement is key. Although the available research on unstageable pressure injuries is growing, there still is considerable need for advancements in the science regarding identification, treatment, and outcomes in critical care patients.

Deep tissue pressure injury (DTPI) is a serious form of pressure injuries. The condition remains invisible for up to 48 hours and then progresses rapidly to full-thickness skin and soft tissue loss. Many other conditions that lead to purple skin can be misidentified as DTPI, making the diagnosis difficult at times. A thorough history exploring exposure to pressure is imperative.

Nutrition is an important component in the prevention and treatment of pressure injuries. Although the point at which insufficient nutrient consumption affects the body's capability to support skin integrity has not been demarcated, what is known is that reduced intake of food and fluids/water and weight loss can increase the risk of developing pressure injuries. Protein and its building blocks, amino acids, are essential for tissue growth and repair during all phases of wound healing. Sufficient macronutrients (carbohydrates, protein, fats, and water) and micronutrients (vitamins and minerals) are vital for the body to support tissue integrity and prevent breakdown.

Patients in critical care units have a multitude of diseases and conditions that contribute to their illness and as such are susceptible to comorbid conditions such as heel pressure injuries. Prevention is a key strategy to avoid heel pressure injury occurrence. Risk factor identification can help a clinician identify those patients at risk for a heel pressure injury requiring timely prevention strategies. The purpose of this article is to raise awareness regarding the critical care patient's vulnerability to heel pressure injuries and strategies that can help avoid their occurrence or expedite their healing if occur.

There are well-documented physiologic changes that occur in the human body during the aging process, such as decreased body fat, decreased muscle mass, cellular senescence, changes in skin pH, decreased metabolism, decreased immune function, vascular changes, altered tissue perfusion, nutritional status changes, and poor hydration. These changes affect skin integrity and wound healing, and raise the risk of pressure-related skin injury. This article discusses aging as a risk factor for pressure injury (PrI). Topics include evidence for advancing age as a significant PrI risk factor, identifying pathophysiologic changes/mechanisms of aging, and specific PrI preventive interventions to consider in older adults.

CRITICAL CARE NURSING
CLINICS OF NORTH AMERICA

SERIES OF RELATED INTEREST

Nursing Clinics of North America
http://www.nursing.theclinics.com

THE CLINICS ARE AVAILABLE ONLINE!
Access your subscription at:
www.theclinics.com

Preface

Pressure Injuries Among Critical Care Patients

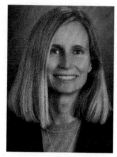

Jenny G. Alderden, PhD, APRN, CCRN, CCNS
Editor

Pressure injuries (PrI), formerly known as pressure ulcers, decubitus ulcers, or bed sores, are one of the oldest documented medical problems. In the nineteenth century, Jean-Martin Charcot, a prominent French physician, described PrI and referred to them as "decubitus ominosus," recognizing the presence of a PrI as an ominous finding. Despite major advances in prevention and treatment, PrI remain a major source of human suffering, particularly in the critical care environment.

PrI prevention and treatment are a team effort. Bedside nurses are often the first critical care clinicians to detect PrI; they are ideally positioned as direct care providers to lead the interdisciplinary care team in PrI prevention and treatment. The care team, composed of critical care nurses, certified wound nurses, providers, nursing assistants, registered dieticians, physical and occupational therapists, pharmacists, and others, works with the patient and their family to plan PrI prevention and/or treatment, continuing to reassess the plan's effectiveness on an ongoing basis.

This current issue of *Critical Care Nursing Clinics of North America* provides up-to-date information to assist critical care nurses in their role as patient advocates and leaders in PrI prevention and treatment. Topics include PrI risk factors, best practice in prevention and treatment, and state-of-the-science information discussing the role of nutrition in PrI prevention and healing. In-depth guidance about more recently identified PrI stages—Unstageable and Deep Tissue Injury—is included, along with special considerations particular to preventing and treating heel PrI with modern medical devices. Finally, this issue details unique PrI prevention and treatment needs among pediatric and older adult populations.

Despite major efforts, PrI incidence in the intensive care unit has increased incrementally over time, notably in the last decade. Given the aging population and ever-increasing severity of illness among critical care patients, the incidence of PrI will likely

Crit Care Nurs Clin N Am 32 (2020) ix–x
https://doi.org/10.1016/j.cnc.2020.09.001
0899-5885/20/© 2020 Published by Elsevier Inc.

ccnursing.theclinics.com

continue to rise. Critical care nurses, armed with state-of-the-science information on Prl prevention and treatment, will play a critical role in reversing the trend.

Jenny G. Alderden, PhD, APRN, CCRN, CCNS
University of Utah College of Nursing
10 South 2000 E
Salt Lake City, UT 84112, USA

E-mail address:
jenny.alderden@utah.edu

Risk Factors for Pressure Injury Development Among Critical Care Patients

Jill Cox, PhD, RN, APN-c, CWOCN[a,b,*]

KEYWORDS

- Pressure injury • Critical care • Risk factors • Intensive care • Pressure ulcer

KEY POINTS

- In order to prevent pressure injuries (PIs) in the critically ill population, accurate determination of pressure injury risk factors is essential.
- Current PI risk assessment tools do not take into consideration the unique risk factors that confront this population.
- Major risk factors that confront the critically ill include age, diabetes, hypotension, mobility, prolonged intensive care unit admission, mechanical ventilation, and vasopressor administration.
- The future of PI risk determination using sophisticated data analytics holds the promise for earlier implementation of targeted PI prevention strategies and will also advance our understanding of the clinical states that may not be modifiable and contribute to unavoidable PIs.

INTRODUCTION

More than 5 million people enter intensive care units (ICUs) across the United States annually for the management of a myriad of critical and life-threatening illnesses and injuries. Top admitting diagnoses to adult ICUs in the United States include respiratory failure with ventilator support, acute myocardial infarction, intracranial hemorrhage/cerebral infarction, and septicemia/severe sepsis.[1,2] Advances in medical technology to treat these conditions have contributed to improved survival rates for many, despite reported increases in the overall severity of illness among critically ill patients, as well as an aging population.[1]

Improved survival may also come with unintended clinical consequences such as the development of a pressure injury (PI). A PI is defined as a localized damage to the skin and underlying soft tissue as a result of pressure or pressure in combination

[a] Rutgers University School of Nursing, 180 University Avenue, Newark, NJ, USA; [b] Englewood Health, Englewood, NJ, USA
* 180 University Avenue, Newark, NJ.
E-mail address: jillcox@sn.rutgers.edu

Crit Care Nurs Clin N Am 32 (2020) 473–488
https://doi.org/10.1016/j.cnc.2020.07.001
0899-5885/20/© 2020 Elsevier Inc. All rights reserved.

with shear usually over a bony prominence or related to a medical or other device.[3] Variability in PI prevalence rates among the critical care population exists globally and ranges between 12% and 24.5%.[4] Attributable health care costs across all settings are now estimated at 26.8 billion dollars annually.[5] Since 2008, pressure injuries have been deemed a never event, with their occurrence in the hospitalized patient subject to reimbursement restrictions from the Centers for Medicare and Medicaid Services.[6] Moreover, PI development has been linked to negative health care outcomes including reduced quality of life, pain, prolonged hospitalizations as well as increases in the risk of mortality, especially in those who have survived a critical illness.[7]

Although substantial evidence supports the efficacy of PI prevention programs in reducing PI,[8,9] no studies have found that the application of these strategies has eliminated all PIs, especially in critically ill patients. In fact, recently reported rates of hospital acquired PIs have been trending upward in the United States. Between the years 2013 and 2016, the mean rate of hospital-acquired PI was reported at 3.6 cases/ 10,000 hospital encounters with an increase in 2016 to 4.8 cases/10,000 hospital encounters. Notably, of these encounters, a 24.6% increase in more severe hospital-acquired PI (stage 3, stage 4, unstageable) was reported between the years 2015 and 2016.[10] In a recent study of hospital-acquired PI rates from the years 2011 to 2016, admission to an ICU was found to be associated with the presence of more severe PIs.[11]

Identification of the appropriate PI risk factors is the first step in successful PI prevention. However, in the critically ill, determination of PI risk is multifactorial and clinically challenging. In a recent review of the empirical literature on PI risk factors in the ICU population, 43 different risk factors across 16 recent studies were identified to be significant predictors of PI development in multivariate analysis, illustrating the multi-etiologic nature of PI risk.[12] PI risk stems from multiple sources when a patient is admitted into an ICU, attributed to the pathophysiologic impacts associated with a critical illness, compounded by potential underlying preexisting comorbid conditions, as well as iatrogenic factors that are often complex, but essential in the ongoing treatment of a critical illness. The purpose of this paper is to examine PI risk factors that have garnered strong empirical support in the critical care population over the past decade.

THE ETIOLOGIC BASIS FOR PRESSURE INJURY DEVELOPMENT

An understanding of how PIs develop is pivotal to our understanding of the factors that contribute to PI risk. An enhanced etiologic framework for PI development has been proposed by Coleman and colleagues[13] and involves an interplay of mechanical forces (pressure, shear, friction) and the ability of the individual to tolerate these forces (**Fig. 1**). The individual's tissue morphology, the physiologic response of the tissue as well as the potential of the tissue to be repaired are all key factors influencing tissue tolerance. Once either the individual's threshold for tissue tolerance or the internal stress produced from mechanical load has been exceeded, the patient is primed for PI occurrence. Tissue ischemia, tissue reperfusion injury, and cell/tissue deformation occur as a result of mechanical load. The individual's ability to mitigate these pathophysiologic changes is a key factor in the development of an impending PI.[14–18]

PRESSURE INJURY RISK ASSESSMENT IN THE INTENSIVE CARE UNIT

Quantifying PI risk through formalized PI risk assessment is considered an essential component of any PI prevention program and is recommended in PI clinical practice guidelines.[3] In the United States, the Braden Scale is the most common PI risk

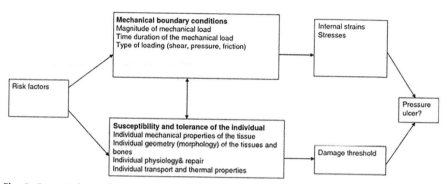

Fig. 1. Factors that influence pressure injury development. (*From* Coleman S, Nixon J, Keen J, et al. A new pressure ulcer conceptual framework. J Adv Nurs. 2014;70(10):2229; with permission.)

assessment scale and is used across all care settings, including the ICU. The Braden scale measures PI risk based on 7 risk factors found on 6 subscales.[19] These subscales include sensory perception, mobility, activity, moisture, nutrition, and friction/shear. Scores range from 6 to 23, with lower scores on the Braden scale indicating greater PI risk.

Tools developed exclusively for use in the ICU setting are scarce. The Jackson/Cubbin scale is one such tool developed for use in the critical care population abroad. The scale measures PI risk based on 12 risk factors, including age, weight, past medical history, mental condition, general skin condition, hemodynamic stability, oxygen requirements, respiratory status, incontinence, mobility, and hygiene.[20,21] Lower scores on this tool equate to higher PI risk.

The predictive validity of PI risk assessment scales among critical care patients has been scrutinized by researchers, with the Braden scale subjected to the most psychometric testing. In order to determine how well risk scales can prospectively predict PI occurrence, a review of the scale's predictive validity must be undertaken. Predictive validity can be determined using 4 key measurements: sensitivity, specificity, predictive value of a negative test (PVN), and predictive value of a positive test (PVP). Sensitivity denotes the scale's ability to predict who is at risk, whereas specificity indicates the tool's ability to predict those not at risk. The PVP and PVN predict who will and will not develop a PI, respectively.[22] In the ICU population, Bergstrom and colleagues[23] were the first to measure the predictive validity of the Braden scale in a sample of 84 adult intensive care patients. **Table 1** outlines the predictive validity for the Braden scale in studies in the critical care population conducted over the past decade.[24–30] Limited studies have evaluated the predictive validity of the Jackson/Cubbin scale; however, in 2 recent investigations, comparing the Jackson/Cubbin scale to the Braden scale in the ICU population, both studies found the Jackson/Cubbin scale to be superior with respect to the scale's predictive validity.[31,32]

Examination of the predictive validity measures of the Braden scale reveals some consistencies among the studies. These include lower specificity and PVP scores, indicating a tendency to overpredict PI risk, a common finding reported among PI risk scales.[22] In the ICU, conceivably all patients will score at risk for PI development; however, the majority will not develop a PI. Clinically, 2 plausible explanations are possible: either the Braden scale score prompted the implementation of appropriate PI prevention strategies, therefore PI develop was averted or conversely, the Braden

Table 1
Predictive validity of the Braden scale in critical care studies

Author	Cut-Off Score	Sensitivity (%)	Specificity (%)	Predictive Value Positive Test (%)	Predictive Value Negative Test (%)
Cox,[24] 2011	18	100	7	20	100
Hyun et al,[25] 2013	18	97	16	10	98
Hyun et al,[26] 2019	ND[a]	67	62	12	96
Jin et al,[27] 2017	ND[a]	77	95	72	95
Ranzani et al,[28] 2016	13	81	66	3.9	99.5
Kim et al[29]	14	92.5	69.8	40.6	97.6
Han et al,[30] 2018	18	63	55	58	60
Adebelli & Korkmaz,[31] 2019	ND[a]	95	75	38	99
Lima-Serrano et al,[32] 2018	12	66.7	55.8	11.7	95

[a] ND: no data provided.

scale failed to differentiate risk magnitude resulting in the implementation of possible unnecessary and potentially costly prevention strategies.[33] It should be noted, however, that in the clinical context of PI risk scale interpretation, the consequences of underprediction would be far more serious than overprediction. Caution is recommended when evaluating the predictive validity of any PI risk assessment scale, as the main purpose of a PI risk assessment scale score is to ascertain PI risk and to drive the implementation of prevention strategies, which can substantially influence PI development.

The total Braden score has been found to be predictive of PI development in multivariate analysis in several studies.[34–38] Less attention, however, has been given to the individual Braden subscales. In clinical practice, the individual subscale scores should be used to guide caregivers toward targeted prevention practices. In studies that have evaluated the Braden subscales as independent variables, the mobility and friction/shear subscales have been found to be predictive in the ICU population.[24,35,37–39]

To date, there are no critical care PI risk assessment scales available that have been validated extensively, thus the need persists for targeted PI risk quantification in this population.

EMPIRICALLY DERIVED PRESSURE INJURY RISK FACTORS

Formalized PI risk assessment assists practitioners in the determination of PI risk for the purpose of implementing prevention practices. In the critical care population, however, there are many unique risk factors not accounted for in PI risk scales that warrant consideration. In recent years, 3 systematic reviews of the literature have been published examining PI risk factors in this population.[12,40,41] Significant predictors of PI development within these reviews included the following: age,[12,40,41] mobility/activity,[40,41] vasopressor infusion,[12,40,41] prolonged ICU admission,[12,41] comorbid conditions (diabetes mellitus,[12,41] cardiovascular disease[12]), hypotension,[12,40,41] prolonged mechanical ventilation,[12,40,41] hemodialysis,[41] and sedation.[41]

Notably across these reviews, commonalities exist. Risk factors with the strongest empirical support include age, diabetes, perfusion (hypotension), mobility, prolonged ICU admission, mechanical ventilation, and vasopressor administration and are the focus of this review. All of these risk factors emerged as significant predictors in 2 or more of these reviews, lending credence to their strength as major PI risk factors in this population that need greater consideration. Moreover, among these risk factors, prolonged ICU admission, use of mechanical ventilation, and use of vasopressors have also been cited in the 2019 International PI Treatment and Practice Guidelines as specific risk factors to consider in the critical care population.[3] These risk factors can be further delineated into 2 broad categories termed intrinsic risk factors, which emerge from physiologic conditions inherent to the patient and extrinsic risk factors, which are forces or situations that are external to the patient and derived from the clinical environment (**Box 1**).

INTRINSIC RISK FACTORS

The risk factors of age, diabetes, mobility, and perfusion (hypotension) can all be categorized as intrinsic, as their basis is rooted in the patient's own physiologic status.

Age

Advancing age has long been recognized as a PI risk factor.[3] In the critical care population, age is cited as one of the most frequently identified predictors of PI development in the empirical literature, identified in 10 studies.[24,34,42–49] The population older than 65 years in the United States grew rapidly for most of the twentieth century, from 3.1 million in 1900 to 35.0 million in 2000 with further expansion for many decades to come, fueled by the baby boom cohort that began turning 65 year old in 2011.[50] When older adults are admitted with a critical illness, they carry with them a complexity and vulnerability not present in the younger population. Factors such as frailty, disability, and multimorbidity are more prevalent with age and increase the risk of adverse outcomes.[51] Age, however, can be a confounding variable when examined in relation to PI risk.[3] As patients age, other conditions associated with aging such as mobility deficits, comorbid conditions that affect tissue oxygenation and perfusion, and nutrition impairments are more likely to occur concomitantly. These factors, when coupled with a critical illness, render the older adult more vulnerable to the potential effects of mechanical load on the skin in addition to a diminished capacity for the tissues to tolerate these forces, both of which are important etiologic factors that contribute to PI.

Box 1

Major pressure injury risk factors among critical care patients

Intrinsic Risk Factors
  Advancing age[24,34,42–49]
  Diabetes mellitus[26,34,44,55]
  Hypotension[37,49,56–61]
  Impaired mobility[24,42,64]

Extrinsic Risk Factors
  Prolonged ICU admission[24,37,42–44,48,59,61,69]
  Mechanical ventilation[26,37,46,48,57,61,72,73]
  Vasopressor agents[24,36,56,57,59,61]

Comorbid Condition: Diabetes Mellitus

According to the Centers for Disease Control and Prevention, diabetes and cardiovascular disease are 2 common chronic diseases that are leading causes of death and disability in the United States.[52] Diabetes results in changes at the microvascular and macrovascular levels. On the microvascular level, diabetes leads to capillary damage and poor perfusion.[53] On the macrovascular level, diabetes is associated with conditions such as peripheral vascular disease, coronary artery disease, and stroke. Cardiovascular disease occurs often times concomitant or as a sequelae of diabetes.[54] Empirically, diabetes mellitus has been found to be a significant predictor of PI development in ICU patient in 4 studies.[26,34,44,55] In the setting of a critical illness, the pathophysiologic effects of diabetes and subsequent cardiovascular disease can exacerbate impaired tissue oxygenation and perfusion, leading to a diminished capacity for the tissues to tolerate pressure, thus contributing to PI development.

Perfusion: Hypotension

Hypotension has emerged as an important PI risk factor in this population and needs greater consideration for its role in PI development. In multiple recent studies, hypotension has emerged as a significant predictor of PI development.[37,49,56–61] Hypotension is an important finding associated with hemodynamic instability. Absolute hypotension is defined as a systolic blood pressure less than 90 mm Hg or mean arterial pressure (MAP) less than 65 mm Hg.[62] Hypotension is the most common presenting manifestation of shock and denotes that perfusion is impaired. In hypotension and shock states, perfusion is shunted from the peripheral circulation in an effort to improve perfusion to the central vital organs. This shunting of blood from the peripheral circulation can compromise tissue perfusion to at-risk anatomic areas such as the sacrum, ischial, and heels. Moreover, impaired tissue perfusion impedes the skin's tolerance for pressure by forcing capillaries to close at lower interface pressures, further contributing to increased risk for PI development.[63]

Mobility

Mobility is defined by the Braden scale as the ability to change or control body position,[19] and activity is defined as one's degree of physical activity such as being ambulatory, bedbound, or chairbound.[19] Mobility impairments frequently in the setting of a critical illness may be so limited such that the patient is completely reliant on caregivers to change position. In one study, lower scores on the Braden mobility subscale score on ICU admission was found to be predictive of PI development.[24] Kaitani and colleagues[64] found infrequent repositioning, measured as the mean daily number of turns, to be predictive of PI development, whereas Tayyib and colleagues[42] identified lower mean hours of patient repositioning to be predictive of PI development.

Repositioning patients is a foundational element of all evidence-based PI prevention programs and is part of routine patient care for ICU patients.[3] However, this population poses unique physiologic and clinical challenges to this basic practice. Impaired mobility among the critically ill can be due to such conditions as hemodynamic instability, unstable spinal fractures, use of sedation, and neuromuscular blocking agents, in addition to iatrogenic factors such as the use of monitoring and treatment devices placed in anatomic areas in which dislodgement is a concern. Surgical procedures that result in an open chest or open abdomen may also alter repositioning practices and in some cases may even preclude repositioning.

To facilitate mobility in the ICU setting, progressive mobility programs have been advocated for over a decade to diminish the systemic adverse effects of immobility.[65–67] In critically ill patients who are not appropriate for progressive mobility or who cannot tolerate regular repositioning, clinical practice guidelines advocate for small weight shifts and microturns as a PI prevention strategy.[3,68] The recognition that there will remain a subset of critically ill patients for which mobility and repositioning practices will need to be severely restricted or suspended also needs consideration in PI risk determination.

EXTRINSIC RISK FACTORS

The risk factors of prolonged ICU admission, mechanical ventilation, and vasopressor administration are extrinsic risk factors, as their roots are associated with factors that occur within the ICU environment.

Prolonged Intensive Care Unit Admission

Prolonged ICU admission is commonly reported as a significant predictor of PI development in this population.[24,37,42–44,48,59,61,69] In the United States, the average length of an ICU admission is reported at 3.8 days; however, this can vary depending on the subtype of ICU and the patient profile.[1] For patients who develop a PI during the ICU admission, the length of the admission usually exceeds this average. For example, Campinili and colleagues[43] in a study of 370 cardiopulmonary ICU patients reported a mean length of stay of 14 days for patients with PI as compared with 4.5 days for those who did not develop a PI. Similarly, Cox in sample of 347 medical/surgical ICU patients reported a mean length of stay in the PI positive group to be 12 days as compared with 3 days for the PI negative group.[24]

Logic would dictate that the longer a patient is cared for in the ICU setting, the greater the chance that the patient will develop a PI. Longer stays in the ICU denotes that the patient is experiencing a higher severity of illness requiring more sophisticated care to stabilize their condition. It is likely that this variable may represent a proxy for the patient's overall burden of critical illness.[12] The identification of ICU length of stay as a significant predictor however usually occurs retrospectively; therefore, it may be more clinically meaningful to identify when in the ICU admission the PI occurred. In studies that have reported the time before PI development, the number of days varies from 3 days to 14 days, with most of the PI occurring in the first 10 days of the ICU admission.[24,42,43,46,55,56,69–71] Therefore many PIs are developing within the early phases of the ICU admission, which correlates with the time period in which the patient is the most hemodynamically unstable and critically ill. Heightened awareness by all caregivers to the increased risk for PI is warranted during this time period.

Mechanical Ventilation

Mechanical ventilation is required by 20% to 40% of all patients in the United States admitted to the ICU and is the most common treatment modality in this setting.[1] Mechanical ventilation is a lifesaving technology that is used in clinical situations in which the patient's own spontaneous respirations are unable to sustain life, leading to impaired gas exchange and subsequent alterations in tissue oxygenation and perfusion. There is strong empirical support for prolonged use of mechanical ventilation as a significant predictor of PI development in this population.[26,37,46,48,57,61,72,73] When identifying mechanical ventilation as a PI risk factor, a few potential clinical scenarios need to be considered. It is plausible that this risk factor may be a proxy for the overall burden of critical illness, suggesting that those who require longer times on mechanical ventilation are the sicker ICU patients. Equally plausible is that this risk factor may be a proxy for immobility, subjecting the patient to increased mechanical load from shear forces as a result of the continuous head of bed elevation required during mechanical ventilation, thus increasing PI risk. Recent studies, however, have examined the role of continuous head elevation in PI development, with findings that do not support continuous head elevation as an independent risk factor for PI development.[61,74,75] Large-scale empirical studies are needed to determine the mechanical effects of continuous head of bed elevation on PI development.

Vasopressor Agents

Vasopressors are medications almost exclusively administered to critical care patients and therefore represent a PI risk factor unique to this population. These agents have emerged in recent empirical investigations as an independent predictor of PI development in critically ill patients cited in 6 studies.[24,36,56,57,59,61]

Vasopressor agents are a powerful class of vasoconstricting medications used to increase MAP commonly in shock states.[76] Commonly used vasopressor agents in clinical practice include norepinephrine, epinephrine, phenylephrine, vasopressin, and dopamine. Although all of these medications share a common purpose to increase MAP, physiologically these medications target different receptors.

A major side effect reported for these medications is hypoperfusion,[76] which can result in deleterious effects to many body systems. Changes to the skin especially to the toes and fingers result in dusky discoloration that can progress to gangrene can occur as a sequelae of these medications in addition to renal compromise, acute limb ischemia in patients with existing peripheral vascular disease as well as renal and mesenteric hypoperfusion.[76]

The pharmacodynamics of these medications suggest that the hypoperfusion induced from these medications may also contribute to changes at bony prominences susceptible to pressure, thus escalating PI risk. However, it remains unknown if the persistent hypotension that dictates the need for the vasopressors, the vasoconstricting properties associated with medication administration, or the overall burden of critical illness experienced by these patients poses the greatest risk for PI development.[57] A paucity of research exists regarding the role of specific vasopressor agents, with 2 recent studies finding norepinephrine and vasopressin emerging as significant predictors.[24,57] Although the evidence is strengthening to support these agents for their role in PI development, continued research into the role of specific vasopressor agents as well as dose and duration of the agents is warranted.

DISCUSSION
Altered Tissue Oxygenation and Perfusion

When considering many of the intrinsic and extrinsic risk factors collectively, a central pathophysiologic premise emerges, one of impaired tissue oxygenation and perfusion. Under normal conditions, the circulatory system delivers adequate oxygen and nutrients to meet the metabolic demands of the body. However, in conditions that commonly affect critically ill patients such as shock states, hypoxia, and hypotension, inadequate cellular oxygen or impaired delivery of oxygen can result in organ dysfunction that can lead to organ failure.[77]

Impaired tissue oxygenation and perfusion have been recognized as important factors to consider when determining PI risk, as these conditions affect overall tissue tolerance, a significant etiologic pathology purported in PI development.[3,13] Among the intrinsically derived risk factors, aging, diabetes, and hypotension all possess altered tissue oxygenation/perfusion as a common pathophysiologic finding. Normal physiologic aging confers a change to one's cardiovascular system, with decreased elasticity and thickening of the vessel walls, leading to impaired exchange of nutrients and wastes.[78] A decrease in vascularity within the dermis as a result of aging impairs the protective function of the skin, thereby contributing to impaired integumentary perfusion.[78] Diabetes mellitus results in changes at both the microvasculature and microvasculature level, with a higher prevalence of cardiovascular disease occurring concomitantly.[79] The presence of these comorbidities in the older population can further intensify tissue oxygenation and perfusion and escalate PI risk. When perfusion is diminished as a result of hypotension, blood flow is shunted away from the periphery to the central circulation, compromising the skin and increasing the risk for ischemic changes. Deeper tissues such as muscle, which is highly vascular, may be more vulnerable to this diminished perfusion, leading to the development of deep tissue pressure injuries (DTPI) and more severe PIs.[14,15] In a study of contributors to DTPIs among 119 ICU patients, hypotension and shock states were found to predictive of the development of a DTPI and increased the likelihood that the DTPI would evolve into a more severe PI (stage 3, stage 4, unstageable).[60]

On examination of the extrinsically derived risk factors, mechanical ventilation and vasopressor administration are treatment factors given to patients to combat clinical situations in which impaired tissue oxygenation and perfusion are the key pathophysiologic determinants. Although vasopressor agents are administered to improve tissue oxygenation/perfusion in patients who are very critically ill and usually in shock, the potent vasoconstriction properties of the medication can worsen these states. Therefore, in patients receiving these medications, impaired tissue oxygenation and perfusion are inherent in both their indication and administration. Mechanical ventilation as a treatment modality is used to improve gas exchange and tissue oxygenation/perfusion in those patients experiencing respiratory failure.[80] In patients requiring mechanical ventilation, improvement in the ventilatory capacity is largely patient dependent on the degree of any underlying pulmonary disease, the cause for the acute respiratory failure as well as the hemodynamic stability of the patient.[80] Therefore, patients requiring prolonged mechanical ventilation may represent a sicker, and less stable subset of critically ill patients, with increased risk for recurring episodes of impaired tissue oxygenation/perfusion, escalating the risk for PI development.

Unavoidable Pressure Injuries: Modifiable and Nonmodifiable Risk Factors

Another important consideration with regard to PI risk, especially in critically ill patients, is the ability to distinguish modifiable risk factors from those that may be nonmodifiable and contribute to unavoidable pressure injuries. The National Pressure Injury Advisory Panel (NPIAP, formerly the National Pressure Ulcer Advisory Panel) defines the unavoidable PI as a PI that develops despite the consistent and appropriate application of PI prevention strategies or if lifesaving modalities take precedence over PI prevention.[81] In 2010, the NPIAP identified potential nonmodifiable risk factors that may be associated with unavoidable PIs and included such risk factors as respiratory instability, arterial insufficiency, vasopressor use, and impaired tissue oxygenation and cardiopulmonary dysfunction due to conditions such as hemodynamic instability, hypotension, heart failure, hypoxemia, and hypotension.[81,82] It is notable that all of these conditions occur in critically ill patients and in many instances are the basis for admission into an ICU.

On examination of the risk factors identified in this review, many could be categorized as nonmodifiable. Acute conditions such as hypotension, depending on the underlying cause, may not be amenable to quick reversal. Similarly, iatrogenic factors such as vasopressor administration and mechanical ventilation, both lifesaving modalities, are immutable and may supersede PI prevention including mobility strategies in hemodynamically unstable patients. Superimposed chronic conditions such as diabetes and cardiac disease may further complicate a critical illness. An awareness that certain clinical scenarios may go beyond the preventive capacity of caregivers is important and assists in identification of PI risk factors that contribute to potentially unavoidable PIs.

In the acute care setting there is a lack of regulatory support for the determination of a PI as unavoidable, which increases an institution's exposure to the financial, quality, and legal consequences. Financial penalties imposed by regulatory agencies,[6,10] concerns regarding the quality of care delivered by nurses[83] as well as the omnipresent threat of litigation[84] once a PI develops are all sequelae of hospital-acquired PIs, even in circumstances in which PI prevention strategies were implemented and suboptimal care was not present. These ramifications create an urgent need to define the unavoidable PI for the acute care setting. Although providing evidence-based PI prevention remains germane to patient care, the first step to defining an unavoidable PI is to strengthen the empirical evidence base and clearly differentiate factors that contribute to PIs that develop as a result of a lack of appropriate evidence-based prevention interventions from those factors that may be prevention immune, thus unmodifiable.

The Future of Pressure Injury Risk Quantification

The future approach to PI risk determination and quantification may look far different from risk assessment of today. Currently, formal PI risk assessment is conducted by the nurse at predetermined time intervals, usually each shift in the ICU. However, PI risk can escalate more frequently as a result of the unstable nature of critical illness. Moreover, as discussed, many risk factors found to be predictive are not captured in PI risk assessment scales, which poses a greater challenge when attempting to determine a patient's level of PI risk.

With the ubiquity of electronic medical records in acute care settings, the feasibility of combining the power of data analytics with the plethora of health information available is within our reach and holds the potential to produce real-time warnings for clinicians regarding changes in clinical condition. In the area of PI risk determination this reality is in the early stages of actualization. Works by Jin and colleagues[27] in the areas of automated PI risk detection and by Alderden and colleagues[85] and Cramer and colleagues[86] using a machine learning approach and artificial intelligence have already been undertaken in this population.

Integration of data analytics into PI risk determination potentially allows the rich source of data from the electronic medical record to discern PI risk based on the unique risk factors that confront critically ill patients. However, automation and the use of sophisticated analytical approaches do impose some known challenges. Spurious mathematical associations are possible, which may produce results that are contrary or illogical to known clinical understanding of a medical condition. Difficulty capturing the appropriate clinical information as a result of how and where particular data elements are housed and coded within the medical record is another concern.[87–89]

SUMMARY

Patients requiring admission to an ICU are complex as a result of their underlying severity of illness, compounded by the need for technologically sophisticated equipment to manage a critical illness and preserve life. As a result, true PI risk determination is equally as complex. Although most ICU patients are found to be at risk for PIs using standardized tools, the empirical literature points to additional factors that escalate PI risk in this population, not quantified in current tools. Important risk factors that need stronger consideration in PI risk determination include the intrinsically derived factors of older age, diabetes mellitus, hypotension, and compromised mobility, as well as the extrinsic factors of longer ICU lengths of stay, prolonged mechanical ventilation, and vasopressor use. The underlying pathophysiologic process inherent in many of these risk factors is altered tissue perfusion and oxygenation, 2 factors that need heightened awareness in PI risk determination when caring for critically ill patients.

With the advent of sophisticated data analytics, automated PI risk prediction may be actualized in the not so distant future. Until this time, current PI risk assessment scales remain, despite the known limitations. Ultimately, improved risk detection holds the possibility for the implementation of earlier and targeted PI prevention strategies in an effort to prevent PIs that are amenable to these strategies. It will also advance our understanding of the clinical states that may not be modifiable and contribute to unavoidable PIs. The ultimate outcome of this knowledge will be an improvement in the quality of care we render to this medically complex population.

DISCLOSURE

The author has nothing to disclose.

REFERENCES

1. Society for Critical Care Medicine. Critical care statistics. Available at: http://www.sccm.org/Communications/Pages/CriticalCareStats.aspx. Accessed November 8, 2019.
2. Barrett ML, Smith MW, Elixhauser A, et al. Utilization of intensive care Services, 2011. Healthcare cost and Ultization Project. 2014. Available at: http://hcup-us.ahrq.gov/reports/statbriefs/sb185-Hospital-Intensive-Care-Units-2011.jsp. Accessed November 8, 2019.
3. National Pressure Injury Advisory Panel, European Pressure Ulcer Advisory Panel and Pan Pacific Pressure Injury Alliance. Prevention and treatment of pressure injuries/ulcers: clinical practice guideline. Emily Haesler. Osborne Park (Western Australia): Cambridge Media; 2019.
4. Chaboyer W, Thalib L, Harbeck E, et al. Incidence and prevalence of pressure injuries in adult intensive care patients: a systematic review. Crit Care Med 2018;46(11):e1074–81.
5. Padula W, Delarmente B. The national cost of hospital acquired pressure injuries in the United States. Int Wound J 2019;16:634–40.
6. Centers for Medicare and Medicaid fact Sheet: never events. Available at: https://downloads.cms.gov/cmsgov/archiveddownloads/smdl/downloads/smd073108.pdf. Accessed October 29, 2019.
7. Lyder C, Wang Y, Metersky M, et al. Hospital-acquired pressure ulcers: results from the national Medicare patient safety monitoring system study. J Am Geriatr Soc 2012;60(9):1603–8.
8. Agency for Healthcare Research and Quality. Preventing pressure ulcers in hospitals: a toolkit for improving quality of care. Rockville (MD): Agency for Healthcare Research and Quality; 2011. Available at: http://www.ahrq.gov/professionals/systems/long-term-care/resources/pressure-ulcers/pressureulcertoolkit/putool3.html. Accessed March 25, 2019.

9. Sullivan N, Schoelles KM. Preventing in-facility pressure ulcers as a patient safety strategy: a systematic review. Ann Intern Med 2013;158(5 Pt 2):410–6.

10. Padula W, Black J, Davidson P, et al. Adverse effects of the Medicare PSI-90 hospital penalty system on revenue-neutral hospital-acquired conditions. J Patient Saf 2020;16(2):e97–102.

11. Kayser S, VanGilder K, Lachenbruch C. Predictors of superficial and severe hospital-acquired pressure injuries: a cross-sectional study using the Internation Pressure Ulcer Prevalence survey. Int J Nurs Stud 2019;89:46–52.

12. Cox J. Pressure injury risk factors in adult critical care patients: a review of the literature. Ostomy Wound Manage 2017;63(11):30–43.

13. Coleman S, Nixon J, Keen J, et al. A new pressure ulcer conceptual framework. J Adv Nurs 2014;70(10):2222–34.

14. Berlowitz D, Brienza D. Are all pressure ulcers the result of deep tissue injury? A review of the literature. Ostomy Wound Manage 2007;53(10):34–8.

15. Oomens CWJ, Bader D, Loerakker S, et al. Pressure induced deep tissue injury explained. Ann Biomed Eng 2015;43(2):297–305.

16. Black J, Brindle C, Honaker J. Differential diagnosis of suspected deep tissue injury. Int Wound J 2015. https://doi.org/10.1111/iwj.12471.

17. Jiang LP, Tu Q, Wang Y. Zhang E Ischemia-reperfusion injury-induced histological changes affecting early stage pressure ulcer development in a rat model. Ostomy Wound Manage 2011;57(2):55–60.

18. Cui F, Pan Y, Xie H, et al. Pressure combined with ischemia/reperfusion injury induces deep tissue injury via endoplasmic reticulum stress in a rat pressure ulcer model. Int J Mol Sci 2016;17(3):284.

19. Bergstrom N, Braden B, Laguzza A, et al. The Braden scale for predicting pressure sore risk. Nurs Res 1987;36(4):205–10.

20. Ahtiala M, Soppi E, Kivimäki R. Critical evaluation of the jackson/cubbin pressure ulcer risk scale - a secondary analysis of a retrospective cohort study population of intensive care patients. Ostomy Wound Manage 2016;62(2):24–33.

21. Jackson C. The revised Jackson/Cubbin pressure area risk calculator. Int Crit Care Nurs 1999;15:169–75.

22. Bolton L. Which pressure ulcer risk assessment scales are valid for clinical use? J Wound Ostomy Continence Nurs 2007;34(4):368–81.

23. Bergstrom N, Demuth P, Braden B. A clinical trial of the Braden scale for predicting pressure sore risk. Nurs Clin North Am 1987;22(2):417–28.

24. Cox J. Predictors of pressure ulcers in adult critical care patients. Am J Crit Care 2011;20(5):364–74.

25. Hyun S, Vermillion B, Newton C, et al. Predictive validity of the braden scale for patients in intensive care units. Am J Crit Care 2013;22(6):514–20.

26. Hyun S, Moffat-Bruce S, Cooper C, et al. Prediction model for hospital-acquired pressure ulcer development: retrospective cohort study. JMIR Med Inform 2019;(3):e13785.

27. Jin Y, Jin T, Lee S. Automated pressure injury risk assessment sytem incorporated int an electronic health record system. Nurs Res 2017;66(6):462–72.

28. Ranzani O, Simpson E, Japiassu A, et al. The challenge of predicting pressure ulcers in critically ill patients: a multicenter cohort study. Ann Am Thorac Soc 2016;13(10):1775–83.

29. Kim E, Lee S, Lee E, et al. Comparison of the predictive validity among pressure ulcer risk assessment scales for surgical ICU patients. Aus J Adv Nurs. 226(4): 87-94. Available at: https://pdfs.semanticscholar.org/e8f9/cd2eaa95fc95442886b82fbc896cc8b2aaed.pdf. Accessed October 13, 2019.

30. Han Y, Jin Y, Lee S. Usefulness of the Braden scale in intensive care units: a study based on electronic health records. J Nurs Care Qual 2018;33(3):238–46.
31. Adibelli S, Korkmaz F. Pressure injury risk assessment in intensive care units: comparison of the reliability and predictive validity of the Braden and Jackson/Cubbin scales. J Clin Nurs 2019. https://doi.org/10.1111/jocn.15054.
32. Lima-Serrano M, González-Méndez MI, Martín-Castaño C. Predictive validity and reliability of the Braden scale for risk assessment of pressure ulcers in an intensive care unit. Med Intensiva 2018;42(2):82–91. English version.
33. Cox J. Predictive power of the Braden Scale for pressure sore risk in adult critical care patients. J Wound Ostomy Continence Nurs 2012;39(6):613–21.
34. Slowikowski G, Funk M. Factors associated with pressure ulcers in patients in a surgical intensive care unit. J Wound Ostomy Continence Nurs 2010;37(6): 619–26.
35. Tescher A, Brando A, Byrne TJO, et al. All at risk patients are not created equal. Analysis of braden pressure ulcer risk scores to identify specific risks. J Wound Ostomy Continence Nurs 2012;39(3):282–91.
36. Tschannen D, Bates O, Talsma A, et al. Patient-specific and surgical characteristics in the development of pressure ulcers. Am J Crit Care 2012;21(2):116–24.
37. Deng X, Yu T, Hu A. Predicting the risk for hospital-acquired pressure ulcers in critical care patients. Crit Care Nurs 2017;37(4):e1–11.
38. Kaewprag P, Newton C, Vermillion, et al. Predictive models for pressure ulcers from intensive care unit electronic records using Bayesian networks. BMC Med Inform Decis Mak 2017;17(Supp 2):81–91.
39. Alderden J, Cummins M, Pepper G, et al. Midrange Braden subscale scores are associated with increased risk for pressure injury development critical care patients. J Wound Ostomy Continence Nurs 2017;4(5):420–8.
40. Alderden J, Rondinelli J. Risk factors for pressure injuries among critical care patients: a systematic review. Int J Nurs Stud 2017;71:97–114.
41. Lima Serrano M, Gonzalez Mendez MI, Carrasco Cebollero FM, et al. Risk factors for pressure ulcer development in intensive care units: a systematic review. Med Intensiva 2017;41(6):339–46.
42. Tayyib N, Coyer F, Lewis P. Saudi Arabian adult intensive care unit pressure ulcer incidence and risk factors: a prospective cohort study. Int Wound J 2016;13(5): 912–9.
43. Campinili T, Conceicao de Gouveia santos V, Strazzieri-Pulido K, et al. Incidence of pressure ulcers in cardiopulmonary intensive carer unit patients. Rev Esc Enferm USP 2015;49:7–13.
44. Nassaji M, Askari Z, Ghorbani R. Cigarette smokikng and risk of pressure ulcers in adult intensive care unit patients. Int J Nurs Prac 2014;20:418–23.
45. O'Brien D, Shanks A, Talsma A, et al. Intraoperative risk factors associated with postoperative pressure ulcers in critically ill patients: a retrospective observational study. Crit Care Med 2013;42(1):40–7.
46. Manzano F, Navarro M, Roldan DM, et al. Pressure ulcer incidence and risk factors in ventilated intensive care patients. J Crit Care 2010;25(3):469–76.
47. Ponchio Pacha H, Lemana Faria J, Aparecido de oliveira K, et al. Pressure ulcers in intensive care units: a case control study. Rev Bras Enferm 2018;71(6): 3027–34.
48. Strazzieri-Pulido KC, S González CV, Nogueira PC, et al. Pressure injuries in critical patients: incidence, patient associated factors, and nursing workload. J Nurs Manag 2019;27:301–10.

49. Soodmand M, Moghadamnia T, Aghaei I, et al. Effects of hemodynamic factors and oxygenation on the incidence of pressure ulcers in the ICU. Adv Skin Wound Care 2019;32:359–64.

50. Roberts AW, Ogunwole SU, Blakeslee L, et al. The population 65 Years and older in the United States: 2016," American Community Survey Reports, ACS-38. Washington, DC: U.S. Census Bureau; 2018.

51. Brummel N, Ferrante L. Integrating geriatric principles into critical care medicine: the time is now. Ann Am Thorac Soc 2018;25(5):518–21.

52. Centers for Disease Control and Prevention. About chronic diseases. 2019. Available at: https://www.cdc.gov/chronicdisease/about/index.htm. Accessed October 24, 2019.

53. Brashers V, Jones R, Huether S. Alterations in hormonal regulation. In: Huether S, McCance K, editors. Understanding pathophysiology. 6th edition. St Louis (MO): Elsevier; 2017. p. 460–89.

54. Brashers V. Alterations in cardiovascular function. In: Huether S, McCance K, editors. Understanding pathophysiology. 6th edition. St Louis (MO): Elsevier; 2017. p. 598–651.

55. Serra R, Caroleo S, Buffone G, et al. Low serum albumin level as an independent risk factor for the onset of pressure ulcers in intensive care unit patients. Int Wound J 2012;11(5):550–3.

56. Bly D, Schallom M, Sona C, et al. A model of pressure, oxygenation, and perfusion risk factors for pressure ulcers in the intensive care unit. Am J Crit Care 2016; 25(2):156–64.

57. Cox J, Roche R. Vasopressors and development of pressure ulcers in adult critical care patients. Am J Crit Care 2015;24(6):501–10.

58. Wilczweski P, Grimm D, Gianakis A, et al. Risk factors associated with pressure ulcer development in critically ill traumatic spinal cord injury patients. J Trauma Nurs 2012;19(1):5–10.

59. El-Marsi J, Zein-El-Dine S, Rita D, et al. Predictors of pressure injuries in a critical care unit in Lebanon. J Wound Ostomy Continence Nurs 2018;45(2):131–6.

60. Kirkland,-Kyhn H, Teleten O, Wilson M. A retrospective, descriptive, comparative study to identify patient variables that contribute to the development of deep tissue injury among patients in intensive care units. Ostomy Wound Manage 2017; 63(2):42–7.

61. Llaurado-Serra M, ulldemolins M, Fenandez-Ballart J, et al. Related factors to semi-recumbent position compliance and pressure ulcers in patients with invasive mechanical ventilation: an observational study(CAPRI study). Int J Nurs Stud 2016;61:198–208.

62. Galeski D, Mikkelsen M. Evaluation of and initial approach to the adult patient with undifferentiated hypotension and shock. 2019. Available at: www.uptodate.com. Accessed October 22, 2019.

63. Pieper B. Pressure ulcers:impact, etiology and classification. In: Bryant R, Nix D, editors. Acute and chronic wounds. 5th edition. St Louis (MO): Elsevier; 2016. p. 124–39.

64. Kaitani T, Tokunaga K, Matsui N, et al. Risk factors related to the development of pressure ulcers in the critical care setting. J Clin Nurs 2010;19:414–21.

65. Vollman KM. Understanding critically ill patient's hemodynamic response to mobilization using the evidence to make it safe and feasible. Crit Care Nurs Q 2013; 36(1):17–27.

66. Topley D. Implementing a mobility program for ICU patients. Am Nurs Today 2015;10(11):15–6.

67. American Association of Critical Care Nurses. Early progressive mobility protocol. 2013. Available at: https://www.aacn.org/docs/EventPlanning/WB0007/Mobility-Protocol-szh4mr5a.pdf. Accessed October 24, 2019.

68. Brindle CT, Malhotra R, O'Rourke S, et al. Turning and repositioning the critically ill patient with hemodynamic instability: a literature review and consensus recommendations. J Wound Ostomy Continence Nurs 2013;40(3):254–67.

69. Cremasco M, Wenzel F, Zanei S, et al. Pressure ulcers in the intensive care unit: the relationship between nursing workload, illness severity, and pressure ulcer risk. J Clin Nurs 2013;22(15–16):2183–91.

70. Efteli E, Gunes U. A prospective, descriptive study of risk factors related to pressure ulcer development among patients in intensive care units. Ostomy Wound Manage 2013;59(7):22–7.

71. Gonzalez-Mendez M, Lima-Serrano M, Martin-Castano C, et al. Incidence and risk factors associated with the development of pressure ulcrs in an intensive care unit. J Clin Nurs 2018;27(5–6):1028–37.

72. Apostolopoulou E, Tselebis A, Terzis K, et al. Pressure ulcer incidence and risk factors in ventilated intensive care patients. Health Sci J 2014;8(3):333–42.

73. Karayurt O, Akyol O, Kilicaslan N, et al. The incidence of pressure ulcers in patients on mechanical ventilation and effects of selected risk factors on pressure ulcer development. Turk J Med Sci 2016;46:1314–22.

74. Schallom M, Dykeman B, Metheny N, et al. Head of bed elevation and early outcomes of gastric reflux, aspiration, and pressure ulcers: a feasibility study. Am J Crit Care 2015;24(1):57–65.

75. Grap MJ, Munro C, Schubert, et al. Lack of association of high backrest with sacral tissue changes in adults receiving mechanical ventilation. Am J Crit Care 2018;27(2):104–13.

76. Manaker S. Us of vasopressors and intropes. 2018. Available at: www.uptodate.com. Accessed October 17, 2019.

77. Ekbal N, Dyson A, Black C, et al. Monitoring tissue perfusion, oxygenation,and metabolism in critically ill patients. Chest 2013;143(6):1799–808.

78. Taffet G. Normal aging. 2019. Available at: www.uptodate.com. Accessed October 15, 2019.

79. Nesto R. Prevalence of and risk factors for coronary heart disease in diabetes mellitus. 2018. Available at: www.uptodate.com. Accessed October 14, 2019.

80. Hyzy R. McSparron, J. Overview of mechanical ventilation. 2018. Available at: www.uptodate.com. Accessed October 17, 2019.

81. Edsberg LE, Langemo, Baharestani MM, et al. Unavoidable pressure injury: state of the science and consensus outcome. J Wound Ostomy Continence Nurs\ 2014;41:313–34.

82. Black J, Edsberg L, Baharestani M. National pressure ulcer advisory panel. pressure ulcers: avoidable or unavoidable. results of the national pressure ulcer advisory panel consensus conference. Ostomy Wound Manage 2011;57(2):24–37.

83. Montalvo I. "The national database of nursing quality IndicatorsTM(NDNQI®)" OJIN: the Online Journal of Issues in nursing. Vol. 12 No. 3, Manuscript 2. 2007. Available at: http://www.nursingworld.org/MainMenuCategories/ANA Marketplace/ANAPeriodicals/OJIN/TableofContents/Volume122007/No3Sept07/NursingQualityIndicators.html. Accessed October 29, 2018.

84. Bennett RG, O'Sullivan J, DeVito EM, et al. The increasing medical malpractice risk related to pressure ulcers in the United States. J Am Geriatr Soc 2000; 48(1):73–81.

85. Alderden J, Pepper G, Wilson A, et al. Predicting pressure injury in critical care patients: a machine learning model. Am J Crit Care 2018;27:461–8.
86. Cramer E, Seneviratne M, Sharifi H. Predicting the incidence of pressure ulcers in the intensive care unit using machine learning. eGEMS J for Electronic Health Data and Methods 2019;7(1):49.
87. Yang S, Stansbury L, Rock P, et al. Linking big data and prediction strategies: tools, pitfalls, and lessons learned. Crit Care Med 2019;47(6):840–8.
88. Hersh W, Weiner M, Embi P, et al. Caveats for the use of operational electronic health record data in comparative effectiveness research. Med Care 2013; 51(8):S30–7.
89. Adibuzzaman M, DeLaurentis P, Hill J, et al. Big data in healthcare-the promises, challenges and opportunities from a research perspective: a case study with a model database. AMIA Annu Symp Proc 2017;2017:384–92.

Best Practice in Pressure Injury Prevention Among Critical Care Patients

Jenny G. Alderden, PhD, APRN, CCRN, CCNS[a],*,
Faygah Shibily, PhD, RN[b], Linda Cowan, PhD, APRN, FNP-BC, CWS[c]

KEYWORDS

- Pressure injury • Prevention • Critical care

KEY POINTS

- Use holistic pressure injury risk assessment to select appropriate preventive interventions.
- Head-to-toe skin and tissue assessment, with particular attention to bony prominences and skin under devices, is a critical aspect of pressure injury prevention aimed at detecting early signs.
- Reposition on an individualized schedule with attention to the individual's support surface, skin status, ability to move in bed, comfort, and activity level.

INTRODUCTION

Pressure injuries (PrIs), formerly called pressure ulcers, are areas of damage to the skin or underlying tissue caused by pressure or a combination of pressure and shear. Individual costs per PrI range from \$12,313 to \$41,326.[1] More than 17,000 lawsuits result from hospital- and facility acquired PrIs annually (second only to wrongful death).[2] In addition to the financial cost, PrIs are a profound source of pain and human suffering.[3,4]

PrIs occur among 6% to 10% of critical care patients[5] and twice as common among intensive care/critical care patients compared with patients admitted to other acute care locations such as medical-surgical units.[6] Therefore, prevention efforts are particularly important in the critical care setting. The purpose of this review article is to describe the current state of the science in PrI prevention among critical care patients. The specific aims are to elucidate the role of PrI risk assessment in prevention and discuss key preventive interventions.

[a] University of Utah College of Nursing, 10 2000 East, Salt Lake City, UT 84112, USA; [b] Faculty of Nursing, King Abdulaziz University, P.O.Box 42828, Jeddah 21551, Saudi Arabia; [c] VISN 8 Patient Safety Center of Inquiry, James A. Haley Veterans Hospital and Clinics, 13000 Bruce B. Downs Boulevard, Tampa, FL 33612, USA
* Corresponding author.
E-mail address: jenny.alderden@utah.edu

Crit Care Nurs Clin N Am 32 (2020) 489–500
https://doi.org/10.1016/j.cnc.2020.08.001
0899-5885/20/© 2020 Elsevier Inc. All rights reserved.

BACKGROUND: PRESSURE INJURY STAGES

PrIs are classified according to stages 1 to 4 based on the suspected level of tissue injury and type of tissue exposed in the wound base.[7] Stage 1 PrI denotes intact skin with nonblanchable redness (that may be reversible), stage 2 refers to partial-thickness loss of skin with exposed dermis, stage 3 PrI refers to full-thickness loss of skin in which fat tissue is visible (extends into subcutaneous tissue but no muscle, tendon, ligament, cartilage, or bone are exposed), and stage 4 PrIs are full-thickness wounds where underlying structures such as fascia, muscle, tendon, ligament, cartilage, or bone are exposed or directly palpable. If intact skin over a bony prominence (or under a medical device) or the wound base in an open PrI exhibits persistent maroon or purple discoloration, the PrI is classified as deep tissue injury. If the depth of an open PrI cannot be evaluated to determine if muscle, fascia, ligament, tendon, or bone may be involved (obscured by eschar or slough), it is considered unstageable until such time as actual tissue depth of injury may be determined. Mucosal membrane PrIs are not staged because mucosal membrane tissue does not have the same structure as other tissue and therefore does not fit the traditional staging system.[8] Furthermore, PrIs due to medical or other devices (such as when the tissue injury may be attributable to laying on a hard tubing) may not occur strictly over bony prominences. For instance, PrIs over the ear may be attributable to mechanical pressure and/or shearing forces from oxygen tubing.[7]

PRESSURE INJURY RISK ASSESSMENT

The PrI risk assessment goal is to identify individuals at risk in order to implement targeted interventions to prevent PrIs, as well as address potentially modifiable risk factors (such as malnutrition).[9] Currently, the National Pressure Injury Advisory Panel (NPIAP) and its sister organizations, the European Pressure Ulcer Advisory Panel (EPUAP) and the Pan Pacific Pressure Injury Alliance (PPPIA), recommend using a structured approach to PrI risk assessment at admission and with changes in patient status.[10] The Braden Scale for Predicting Pressure Ulcer Risk (Braden Scale) is the structured risk assessment most commonly used in the critical care setting. The Braden Scale was first published in 1987 by Bergstrom, Demuth, and Braden.[11,12] The Braden Scale total score sums the values of 6 subscales: moisture, mobility, activity, friction and shear, nutrition, and sensory perception; patients are categorized from very high risk ($\leq$9) to low risk (19–23).[11] Since 1987, the Braden Scale has remained largely unchanged in both the risk factors it attempts to identify and the scoring and cutoff points.

Studies conducted among critical care patients demonstrated the Braden Scale lacks predictive validity in that population because it tends to identify most critical care patients as "high risk" (low specificity, high sensitivity).[13] Because the Braden Scale total score lacks the predictive validity needed to guide more intense preventive efforts in the intensive care setting, some experts also recommend using Braden Scale *subscale* scores (moisture, activity, mobility, nutrition, friction and shear, and sensory perception) to guide care planning.[14] For example, moist skin can be addressed by keeping skin dry, applying barrier creams, continence management, etc., and patients with inadequate nutritional intake will benefit from efforts to optimize nutrition status and address nutritional deficits. However, the Braden Scale nutrition is an inaccurate measure of nutrition status likely due to a high degree of subjectivity.[15] Moreover, a recent study examining changes in Braden subscale scores over time showed patients with mild to moderate risk (as opposed to high-risk Braden subscale scores) were at increased risk for PrI development in all subscale categories except friction and shear.[16] More study is needed to identify critical care patients at highest risk for PrIs, elucidating the relationship between specific Braden Scale subscales and risk in the critical care setting.

Instead of relying on the total score of a risk assessment score alone, the NPIAP, EPUAP, and PPPIA recommend basing risk-based prevention on a holistic approach to PrI risk assessment. Holistic approaches include structured risk assessment total score, subscale scores, and careful attention to other relevant factors unaccounted for in risk assessment tools and/or unique to a care setting or specific patient population.[10] In the critical setting, altered perfusion (inadequate delivery of oxygen-rich blood to the tissue) is particularly relevant and should be considered in PrI risk assessment and associated care planning. Inadequate perfusion refers to the inadequate delivery of oxygen-rich blood to the tissue, resulting in tissue hypoxia and potential PrI development.[17] Inadequate perfusion commonly occurs among critical care patients receiving vasopressors due to a combination of peripheral vasoconstriction and the disease process requiring the use of a vasopressor.[18] Nonpulsatile blood flow— such as in patients receiving extracorporeal membrane oxygenation or patients undergoing some types of cardiac surgery—is another potential perfusion-related PrI risk factor encountered in critical care.

In addition to perfusion, other PrI risk factors commonly identified among critical care patients worth consideration in care planning include older age, hemodynamic instability, ventilator status, multiorgan failure, surgical procedures, and specific disease states. Advanced age confers risk due to a combination of physiologic changes associated with aging and comorbid conditions more prevalent among older people.[19–25] Activity limitations (also an included factor in the Braden Scale)[11] is associated with risk for PrIs due to a combination of general deconditioning and the patient's inability to independently reposition to redistribute pressure.[26,27] Although few studies have identified specific surgical risk factors among critical care patients,[28] surgical-critical care populations have higher overall PrI incidence compared with patients admitted to other types of critical care units.[5] Finally, among critical care patients, other PrI risk factors include diagnoses of diabetes,[21] renal failure,[21,29] heart disease,[18,21,26] and/or vascular disease.[24]

Ultimately, PrI risk assessment exists to help nurses and other members of the multidisciplinary health care team select effective preventive interventions, including the frequency of skin assessment and repositioning along with other interventions described in more detail later. Some interventions relate directly to the specific risk factors (eg, eliminating moisture for moist skin), whereas other interventions are allotted based on the patient's estimated overall level of risk, and this includes the clinician's holistic assessment of risk based on each patient's unique profile and intersecting risk factors.

PREVENTIVE INTERVENTIONS

The following section summarizes preventive interventions in the following domains: skin and tissue assessment and preventive skin care, repositioning, nutrition, support surfaces, early mobilization, and special populations.[10] Recommendations in each domain are summarized in **Box 1**.

Skin and Tissue Assessment and Preventive Skin Care

Skin status broadly refers to the skin's overall condition as well as the presence of previous skin problems such as a chronic wound or a prior PrI.[10] The presence of an existing PrI is associated with increased risk for additional, subsequent PrI development.[30]

Box 1
Pressure injury prevention interventions by domain

Skin and Tissue Assessment
- Conduct head-to-toe skin inspection on an individualized schedule
- Assess for areas of redness, swelling, or change in skin temperature or texture
- Offload skin with changes in color, temperature, or texture
- Carefully assess skin under medical devices and offload pressure if skin changes are noted

Preventive Skin Care
- Keep skin clean and dry
- Moisturize excessively dry skin
- Use moisture barrier creams on areas with persistent moisture exposure
- Avoid vigorous scrubbing motions
- If a patient develops incontinence-associated dermatitis, consider use of a urinary catheter or fecal management system
- Use multilayered silicone foam dressings on heels and bony prominences in high-risk patients, unless contraindicated

Repositioning
- Routinely reposition patients on individualized schedules
- Ensure that a sufficient turn angle is reached to allow tissue offloading
- Avoid friction and shearing forces
- If clinically feasible, position the head of bed as flat as possible
- Use heel floatation unless contraindicated
- Consider cues to remind nurses and other caregivers to adhere to the repositioning schedule

Nutrition
- Screen all patients for nutrition risk using a validated tool
- Collaborate with a Registered Dietician to develop a nutrition plan for at-risk patients

Support Surfaces (beds)
- Use an industry-standard support surface
- Ensure the support surface is large enough to allow the patient to turn comfortably
- Continuous rotation features do not replace manual turning

Early Mobilization
- Unless contraindicated, initiate early mobilization
- Limit time spent in a chair to 2 hours or less at a time

Stage 1 PrIs are at particular risk for deterioration into a more severe stage[31–33]; in critical care patients, stage 1 worsens into stage 2 or more severe stages approximately one-third of the time.[33] Also, other alterations in skin status including excessive moisture, dryness, irritation, and inflammation are all associated with increased susceptibility to PrI.[10,34]

Head-to-toe skin and tissue assessment with particular attention to bony prominences and skin under devices is a critical aspect of PrI prevention aimed at detecting early signs. The skin assessment is conducted visually and via touch (assessing skin temperature and texture); the timing and frequency is based on an individual's PrI risk. The major focus of the head-to-toe skin assessment is to identify areas of erythema (redness), swelling, or a change in skin temperature or texture.[35] Blanchable erythema refers to skin redness becoming white when pressure is applied and then reddens when pressure is relieved, whereas in nonblanchable erythema, the redness persists when pressure is applied—nonblanchable erythema is a stage 1 PrI. Both stage 1 PrI and blanchable erythema should be offloaded as soon as possible to prevent additional, more severe tissue damage.[34] In individuals with darker skin, where erythema is less noticeable or may not be visible, edema and changes in temperature and texture are critical assessment parameters indicating areas of the body requiring immediate offloading.[36] Finally, in addition to visual assessment and tactile assessment, objective measures of skin status (such as thermography and measures of subepidermal moisture)[35,37] may also be used in nursing skin assessment.

Along with offloading pressure on areas of skin with redness or alterations in temperature or texture, skin protection and integrity promotion remain imperative. In the critical care environment, maintaining skin integrity includes careful attention to skin hygiene and may include managing skin conditions, such as incontinence-associated dermatitis. Managing skin hygiene includes keeping the skin clean, dry, and hydrated, while also avoiding alkaline skin products and using a moisture barrier cream in patients with persistent exposure to moisture.[10,38] It is vital to avoid vigorous scrubbing when cleansing, because the back and forth motion may damage the skin via friction.[39] Incontinence-associated dermatitis, inflammation or erosion of the skin associated with exposure to urine or feces, is associated with increased risk for PrIs.[39] Incontinence-associated dermatitis should be managed by preventing further contact between the skin and body fluids, which may require the use of a urinary catheter or fecal management device.[40] Gentle skin cleansing, moisturization with an emollient, and application of skin protectant (barrier creams) are also important.[40]

Some evidence suggests the use of prophylactic multilayered silicone foam dressings applied to bony prominences, such as the sacrum and heels, may be useful for PrI prevention in certain situations.[41] Use of a prophylactic dressing does not preclude the importance of regular skin assessment; therefore, it is important to select a dressing easily peeled back—transparent options are also available. Although generally useful, prophylactic dressings may not be appropriate for patients who experience frequent incontinence because moisture and body fluids may become trapped in the dressing.

Repositioning

Repositioning to offload, or redistribute, pressure is a mainstay of PrI prevention. PrIs are caused by a combination of tissue deformation, inflammation, and ischemia[10]— tissue deformation, an essential component of the cause of PrI,[42] can be prevented or ameliorated with pressure redistribution. The NPIAP recommends repositioning all patients on an individualized schedule with attention to the individual's support surface, skin status, ability to move in bed, comfort, and activity level.[10] In 2014, Manzano and colleagues[43] compared 2- and 4-hour repositioning schedules among critical care patients undergoing mechanical ventilation and determined there was no significant difference in PrI incidence between the 2 groups. Similarly, Bergstrom and colleagues[44] found no significant difference in PrI incidence among long-term care residents assigned to 2-, 3-, or 4-hour repositioning schedules among older people in a long-term care setting. The adequacy of a repositioning schedule should be routinely checked using careful skin assessment; persistent redness on a body part indicates the patient should be repositioned more often.[10]

During repositioning, ensuring a sufficient turn angle is reached in order to offload a section of the body can be challenging; for hard-to-position people, wedges may be useful to enable turn angles.[45] Avoid excessive turn angles; in one study, patients repositioned in a side-lying position were at increased risk for PrIs compared with patients who were positioned at a 30° turn angle.[46] Avoid friction (sliding of the skin and a surface against each other) and shearing forces (pushing one part of the body in one direction where the skin tissue moves in the opposite direction) that can damage tissue, and this may be achieved by lifting the patient (or using a mechanical lift) to avoid dragging a patient across the bed surface.[47] If clinically feasible, the head of bed position should be kept as flat as possible to avoid increased interface pressure at the sacrum.[10] However, evidence for flatter head of bed positions is inconsistent, and risk for PrI needs to be balanced against other considerations relevant in the critical care population such as risk for ventilator-associated pneumonia.[48] Heel floatation, using pillows or a heel floatation boot, effectively offloads the heel and should be applied unless contraindicated.

Some critical care patients experience hemodynamic instability with repositioning, hence the expression "too unstable to turn." However, in most cases, even hemodynamically unstable patents can be safely turned using a slow, incremental approach.[49] For example, adjusting the patient's position very slightly by putting a flat pillow under the trunk, hip, and thigh on one side could achieve a slight position change of 15°, which could be alternated with the other side in 1 to 2 hours. Currently, no studies have demonstrated which degree of turn angle adequately offloads tissue, but consensus determines even a very small turn is likely better than no turn at all. For patients completely intolerant of activity, interventions such as heel elevation, passive limb movements, and small weight shifts may be possible and should be trialed.[49] The NPIAP recommends attempting repositioning unstable patients at least every 8 hours, to assess tolerance. However, this recommendation may be altered in cases where the risks of repositioning in terms of hemodynamic stability outweigh the potential skin benefits.[10]

Repositioning schedules can be difficult to maintain due to competing priorities and caregivers' cognitive load (ie, in a busy intensive care unit, it is easy to forget to turn a patient). Cueing systems, such as musical chimes occurring at regular intervals or wearable sensors, are both effective ways to remind nurses and other caregivers on a consistent and individualized basis.[50,51]

Nutrition

Nutrition and hydration closely relate to skin health.[10,52] However, there is limited high-quality evidence pertaining to nutritional status and interventions to prevent PrIs, due in part to inconsistency in defining and measuring nutrition and hydration.[53] Although commonly used to assess nutrition related to PrI risk, the Braden Scale's nutrition subscale insufficiently measures nutrition status due to a high degree of subjectivity.[15,54] Instead, the NPIAP recommends screening for nutritional risk using the Mini Nutritional Assessment or another validated tool.[10,55] Critical Care patients with nutritional risk should be followed closely by a Registered Dietitian in collaboration with the multidisciplinary care team.

Support Surfaces (Beds and Mattresses)

Selecting an appropriate support surface, or bed (and mattress) type, imperatively affects PrI prevention in the critical care population. A full discussion of the different types of support surfaces is outside the scope of this article; however, the following recommendations from the National Pressure Injury Prevention Coalition apply.[10] First, the support surface should be tested to ensure the surface (bed) meets industry standards. Second, the surface should allow enough room for the patient to turn comfortably; larger patients may require a specialized bariatric bed. Third, continuous lateral rotation features should not be considered a replacement for manual turning and repositioning, as no current evidence indicates continuous lateral rotation therapy, a lung-protective strategy, adequately offloads pressure on the skin.[56] Finally, the use of alternating pressure mattresses or mattress overlays likely facilitates PrI prevention, although more information is needed to determine the magnitude of the effect.[57]

Early Mobilization

Early mobilization among critical care patients improves functional status across a range of outcomes.[58] Although mobilization is beneficial, the relationship between early mobilization and PrI development is inconsistent, with some studies showing increased PrI incidence[59] or no change[60] and others finding decreased PrI incidence.[61] The NPIAP recommends early mobility as a PrI prevention strategy[10] with the caveat that excessive time spent sitting in a chair without repositioning should be avoided. One study determined limiting the amount of time spent in a chair to 2 hours or less at a time reduced the incidence of PrIs compared with longer durations of time spent in a chair.[62]

Special Populations

Some special populations, such as older patients, obese patients, and patients with spinal cord injury, require special PrI prevention considerations. Older adults experience increased risk for PrIs due to age-related changes, including thinning skin, decreased subcutaneous tissue, flattening of the dermoepidermal junction (decrease in rete ridges), structural depletion of collagen fibers in the dermis, vertical capillary loops loss, and elasticity loss.[63] Along with aging-related skin changes, older people may also experience reduced mobility and/or reduced sensory perception. Results from a systematic review of risk factors for hospital-acquired PrIs among critical care patients determined older age is an independent risk factor in this population.[5] Nurses caring for older patients should individualize repositioning and skin inspection schedules in this population, recognizing older people with reduced sensory perception may not recognize when skin is exposed to excessive pressure.

Obese patients also require special consideration in PrI prevention. It is necessary to choose a bed enabling the patient to have enough room to move freely from side to side without wedging themselves against a side rail.[64] Skin folds resulting from obesity may become moist or macerated, increasing risk for PrIs, and should be kept clean and dry.[64] Safe patient handling and mobility equipment such as ceiling mounted or floor-based lifting devices are essential in this population for caregiver safety, simultaneously avoiding the risk of exposing the patient to friction and/or shearing forces.[64]

Patients with spinal cord injury experience increased risk for PrIs for a variety of reasons. Immobility and altered sensory perception both potentially expose patients to pressure and autonomic changes in spinal cord injury affect skin perfusion.[10] Nurses should carefully conduct frequent skin assessment in this population, especially under stabilization devices (eg, cervical collars, traction) used for trauma patients with actual or potential spinal cord injuries.[65,66] The initial stabilization period is a particularly vulnerable time for patients with spinal cord injury; in one study conducted among trauma patients with spinal cord injury, nearly half (45%) of PrIs developed within 48 hours of hospitalization.[67] However, even after the initial stabilization period patients with any level of spinal cord injury remain at risk. In a recent study, long-term care patients with paraplegia were *more* likely to develop PrIs than patients with quadriplegia—underscoring the importance of careful PrI prevention efforts in all spinal cord injured patients.

SUMMARY

PrI prevention is an ongoing effort in the critical care environment, requiring careful attention from nurses and other members of the multidisciplinary team. The selection of appropriate preventive interventions requires a holistic approach, including the evaluation of the individual patient's unique risk factors. To be effective, risk assessment and selection of appropriate interventions must be conducted frequently to keep pace with dynamic changes in patient status, often a challenge in the critical care environment. It remains vital to continue an ongoing assessment of the adequacy of preventive interventions via careful skin assessment to identify potential problem areas or early stage PrIs.

ADDITIONAL RESOURCES

The current article summarizes best practice in preventive interventions in the following domains: skin and tissue assessment and preventive skin care, repositioning, nutrition, support surfaces, early mobilization, and special populations. A free, quick-reference guide based on the NPIAP 2019 international prevention and treatment guidelines is available at https://guidelinesales.com/store/ViewProduct.aspx?id=15037164.

DISCLOSURE

The authors have nothing to disclose.

REFERENCES

1. Bysshe T, Gao Y, Heaney-Huds K, et al. Estimating the additional hospital inpatient cost and mortality associated with selected hospital-acquired conditions. Agency for Healthcare Research and Quality Web site. Available at: https://www.ahrq.gov/professionals/quality-patient-safety/pfp/haccost2017.html. Accessed June 22, 2019.
2. Preventing pressure ulcers in hospitals. Agency for healthcare research and quality web site. Available at: https://www.ahrq.gov/professionals/systems/hospital/pressureulcertoolkit/putool1.html. Accessed June 20, 2019.
3. Ahn H, Stechmiller J, Horgas A. Pressure ulcer-related pain in nursing home residents with cognitive impairment. Adv Skin Wound Care 2013;26(8):375–80 [quiz: 381–2].
4. Woo KY, Sears K, Almost J, et al. Exploration of pressure ulcer and related skin problems across the spectrum of health care settings in Ontario using administrative data. Int Wound J 2017;14(1):24–30.
5. Alderden J, Rondinelli J, Cummins M, et al. Risk factors for pressure injuries among critical care patients: a systematic review. Int J Nurs Stud 2017;71:97–114.
6. Baumgarten M, Margolis DJ, Localio AR, et al. Extrinsic risk factors for pressure ulcers early in the hospital stay: a nested case-control study. J Gerontol A Biol Sci Med Sci 2008;63(4):408–13.
7. Edsberg LE, Black JM, Goldberg M, et al. Revised National pressure ulcer advisory panel pressure injury staging system: revised pressure injury staging system. J Wound Ostomy Continence Nurs 2016;43(6):585–97.
8. NPUAP position statement on staging — 2017 clarifications. National Pressure Ulcer Advisory Panel. 2017. Available at: https://cdn.ymaws.com/npuap.org/resource/resmgr/npuap-position-statement-on-.pdf. Accessed April 8, 2020.
9. Stechmiller JK, Cowan L, Whitney JD, et al. Guidelines for the prevention of pressure ulcers. Wound Repair Regen 2008;16(2):151.
10. European Pressure Ulcer Advisory Panel, National Pressure Injury Advisory Panel, Pan Pacific Pressure Injury Alliance. Prevention and treatment of pressure

ulcers/injuries: clinical practice guideline. In: Haesler E, editor. The international guideline. EPUAP/NPIAP/PPPIA; 2019.

11. Bergstrom N, Braden BJ, Laguzza A, et al. The Braden Scale for predicting pressure sore risk. Nurs Res 1987;36(4):205–10.

12. Bergstrom N, Demuth PJ, Braden BJ. A clinical trial of the Braden scale for predicting pressure sore risk. Nurs Clin North Am 1987;22:417–28.

13. Cox J. Predictive power of the Braden Scale for pressure sore risk in adult critical care patients: a comprehensive review. J Wound Ostomy Continence Nurs 2012; 39(6):613–21 [quiz: 622–3].

14. Ayello EA. Using pressure ulcer risk assessment tools in care planning. Lecture presented at: Excelsior College School of Nursing. Available at: https://www.ahrq.gov/sites/default/files/wysiwyg/professionals/systems/hospital/pressure_ulcer_prevention/webinars/webinar5_pu_riskassesst-tools.pdf. Accessed October 30, 2019.

15. Cowan L, Garven C, Kent C, et al. How well does the Braden nutrition subscale Agree with the VA nutrition classification scheme related to pressure ulcer risk? Fed Pract 2016;33(12):12–7.

16. Alderden J, Cummins M, Pepper GA, et al. Mid-range Braden subscale scores are associated with increased risk for pressure injury among ICU patients. J Wound Ostomy Continence Nurs 2017;44(5):420.

17. Coleman S, Nixon J, Keen J, et al. A new pressure ulcer conceptual framework. J Adv Nurs 2014;70(10):2222–34.

18. Cox J, Roche S. Vasopressors and development of pressure ulcers in adult critical care patients. Am J Crit Care 2015;24(6):501–10.

19. Tayyib N, Coyer F, Lewis P. Saudi Arabian adult intensive care unit pressure ulcer incidence and risk factors: a prospective cohort study. Int Wound J 2015. https://doi.org/10.1111/iwj.12406.

20. Slowikowski GC, Funk M. Factors associated with pressure ulcers in patients in a surgical intensive care unit. J Wound Ostomy Continence Nurs 2010;37(6): 619–26.

21. O'Brien DD, Shanks AM, Talsma A, et al. Intraoperative risk factors associated with postoperative pressure ulcers in critically ill patients: a retrospective observational study. Crit Care Med 2014;42(1):40–7.

22. Manzano F, Navarro MJ, Roldán D, et al. Pressure ulcer incidence and risk factors in ventilated intensive care patients. J Crit Care 2010;25(3):469–76.

23. Eachempati SR, Hydo LJ, Barie PS. Factors influencing the development of decubitus ulcers in critically ill surgical patients. Crit Care Med 2001;29(9):1678–82.

24. Nijs N, Toppets A, Defloor T, et al. Incidence and risk factors for pressure ulcers in the intensive care unit. J Clin Nurs 2009;18(9):1258–66.

25. Alderden J, Pepper G. Critical care patients with special needs: care of the older adult. In: Hartjes TJ, editor. AACN core curriculum for critical care nursing. Annapolis (MD): Elsevier; 2018. p. 732–40.

26. Cox J. Predictors of pressure ulcers in adult ICU patients. Am J Crit Care 2011; 20(5):364–75.

27. Sayar S, Turgut S, Dogan H, et al. Incidence of pressure ulcers in intensive care unit patients at risk according to the Waterlow scale and factors influencing the development of pressure ulcers. J Clin Nurs 2009;18(5):765–74.

28. Tschannen D, Bates O, Talsma A, et al. Patient-specific and surgical characteristics in the development of pressure ulcers. Am J Crit Care 2012;21(2):116–25.

29. Frankel H, Sperry J, Kaplan L. Risk factors for pressure ulcer development in a best practice surgical intensive care unit. Am Surg 2007;73(12):1215–7.

30. Baumgarten M, Margolis D, van Doorn C, et al. Black/White differences in pressure ulcer incidence in nursing home residents. J Am Geriatr Soc 2004;52(8): 1293–8.

31. Nixon J, Cranny G, Bond S. Skin alterations of intact skin and risk factors associated with pressure ulcer development in surgical patients: a cohort study. Int J Nurs Stud 2007;44(5):655–63.

32. Demarre L, Verhaeghe S, Van Hecke A, et al. Factors predicting the development of pressure ulcers in an at-risk population who receive standardized preventive care: secondary analyses of a multicenter randomized controlled trial. J Adv Nurs 2015;71(2):391–403.

33. Alderden J, Zhao YL, Zhang Y, et al. Outcomes associated with stage 1 pressure injuries: a retrospective cohort study. Am J Crit Care 2018;27(6):471–6.

34. Compton F, Hoffmann F, Hortig T, et al. Pressure ulcer predictors in ICU patients: nursing assessment versus objective parameters. J Wound Care 2008;17(10): 417–24.

35. Cox J, Kaes L, Martinez M, et al. A prospective, observational study to assess the use of thermography to predict progression of discolored intact skin to Necrosis among patients in skilled nursing facilities. Ostomy Wound Manage 2016;62(10): 14–33.

36. Farid KJ, Winkelman C, Rizkala A, et al. Using temperature of pressure-related intact discolored areas of skin to detect deep tissue injury: an observational, retrospective, correlational study. Ostomy Wound Manage 2012;58(8):20–31.

37. Park S, Kim CG, Ko JW. The use of sub-epidermal moisture measurement in predicting blanching erythema in jaundice patients. J Wound Care 2018;27(5): 342–9.

38. Ananthapadmanabhan KP, Moore DJ, Subramanyan K, et al. Cleansing without compromise: the impact of cleansers on the skin barrier and the technology of mild cleansing. Dermatol Ther 2004;17(Suppl 1):16–25.

39. Park KH, Kim KS. Effect of a structured skin care regimen on patients with fecal incontinence: a comparison cohort study. J Wound Ostomy Continence Nurs 2014;41(2):161–7.

40. Gray M, Bliss DZ, Doughty DB, et al. Incontinence-associated dermatitis: a review. J Wound Ostomy Continence Nurs 2007;34(1):45–54 [quiz: 55–6].

41. Kalowes P, Messina V, Li M. Five-layered soft silicone foam dressing to prevent pressure ulcers in the intensive care unit. Am J Crit Care 2016;25(6):e108–19.

42. Gefen A. Bioengineering models of deep tissue injury. Adv Skin Wound Care 2008;21(1):30–6.

43. Manzano F, Colmenero M, Pérez-Pérez AM, et al. Comparison of two repositioning schedules for the prevention of pressure ulcers in patients on mechanical ventilation with alternating pressure air mattress. Intensive Care Med 2014; 40(11):1679–87.

44. Bergstrom N, Horn SD, Rapp MP, et al. Turning for Ulcer Reduction: a multisite randomized clinical trial in nursing homes. J Am Geriatr Soc 2013;61(10): 1705–13.

45. Latimer S, Chaboyer W, Gillespie BM. The repositioning of hospitalized patients with reduced mobility: a prospective study. Nurs Open 2015;2(2):85–93.

46. Moore Z, Cowman S, Posnett J. An economic analysis of repositioning for the prevention of pressure ulcers. J Clin Nurs 2013;22(15–16):2354–60.

47. Gould L, Abadir P, Brem H, et al. Chronic would repair and healing in older adults: current status and future research. Wound Repair Regen 2015;23(1):1–13.

48. Niël-Weise BS, Gastmeier P, Kola A, et al. An evidence-based recommendation on bed head elevation for mechanically ventilated patients. Crit Care 2011; 15(2):R111.

49. Brindle C, Malhotra R, O'Rouke S, et al. Turning and repositioning the critically ill patient with hemodynamic instability: a literature review and consensus recommendations. J Wound Ostomy Continence Nurs 2013; 40(3):254–67.

50. Yap TL, Kennerly SM, Simmons MR, et al. Multidimensional team-based intervention using musical cues to reduce odds of facility-acquired pressure ulcers in long-term care: a paired randomized intervention study. J Am Geriatr Soc 2013;61(9):1552–9.

51. Pickham D, Berte N, Pihulic M, et al. Effect of a wearable patient sensor on care delivery for preventing pressure injuries in acutely ill adults: a pragmatic randomized clinical trial (LS-HAPI study). Int J Nurs Stud 2018;80:12–9.

52. Dorner B, Posthauer ME, Thomas D. The role of nutrition in pressure ulcer prevention and treatment: National pressure ulcer advisory panel white paper. In: National Pressure Ulcer Advisory Panel. 2009. Available at: https://pdfs.semanticscholar.org/b265/79036000570d935958b1a39bb421380c82e7.pdf. Accessed December 27, 2019.

53. Posthauer ME, Banks M, Dorner B, et al. The role of nutrition for pressure ulcer management. National Pressure Ulcer Advisory Panel, European Pressure Ulcer Advisory Panel, and Pan Pacific Pressure Injury Alliance White Paper. Adv Skin Wound Care 2015;28(4):175–88.

54. Phillips W, Hershey M, Willcutss K, et al. The effectiveness of the Braden scale as a tool for identifying nutrition risk. J Acad Nutr Diet 2018;118(3):385–7, 389-391.

55. Vellas B, Guigoz Y, Garry PJ, et al. The Mini Nutritional Assessment (MNA) and its use in grading the nutritional state of elderly patients. Nutrition 1999;15(2): 116–22.

56. Kirschenbaum L, Azzi E, Sfeir T, et al. Effect of continuous lateral rotational therapy on the prevalence of ventilator-associated pneumonia in patients requiring long-term ventilatory care. Crit Care Med 2002;30(9):1983–6.

57. Shi C, Dumville JC, Cullum N. Support surfaces for pressure ulcer prevention: a network meta-analysis. PLoS One 2018;13(2):e0192707.

58. Adler J, Malone D. Early mobilization in the intensive care unit: a systematic review. Cardiopulm Phys Ther J 2012;23(1):5–13.

59. Dammeyer J, Dickinson S, Packard D, et al. Building a protocol to guide mobility in the ICU. Crit Care Nurs Q 2013;36(1):37–49.

60. Wood W, Tschannen D, Trotsky A, et al. A mobility program for an inpatient acute care medical unit. Am J Nurse 2014;114(10):34–40 [quiz: 41–2].

61. Klein K, Mulkey M, Bena JF, et al. Clinical and psychological effects of early mobilization in patients treated in a neurologic ICU: a comparative study. Crit Care Med 2015;43(4):865–73.

62. Gebhardt K, Bliss MR. Preventing pressure sores in orthopaedic patients – is prolonged chair nursing detrimental? J Tissue Viability 1994;4(2):51–4.

63. Mine S, Fortunel NO, Pageon H, et al. Aging alters functionally human dermal papillary fibroblasts but not reticular fibroblasts: a new view of skin morphogenesis and aging. PLoS One 2008;3:e4066.

64. Mathison CJ. Skin and wound care challenges in the hospitalized morbidly obese patient. J Wound Ostomy Continence Nurs 2003;30(2):78–83.

65. Grigorian A, Sugimoto M, Joe V, et al. Pressure ulcer in trauma patients: a higher spinal cord injury level leads to higher risk. J Am Coll Clin Wound Spec 2017; 9(1–3):24–31.

66. Jackson D, Sarki AM, Betteridge R, et al. Medical device-related pressure ulcers: a systematic review and meta-analysis. Int J Nurs Stud 2019;92:109–20.

67. Ham HW, Schoonhoven LL, Schuurmans MM, et al. Pressure ulcer development in trauma patients with suspected spinal injury; the influence of risk factors present in the emergency department. Int Emerg Nurs 2017;30:13–9.

Best Practices in Pressure Injury Treatment

Andrea L. Roufogalis, BSN, CWON,
Melissa L. Hutchinson, DNP, ARNP-CNS, CCNS, CWCN-AP, CCRN*

KEYWORDS

- Interprofessional • Team composition • Pressure injury • Treatment

KEY POINTS

- Identify factors that impair wound healing.
- Describe signs and symptoms indicating a wound infection.
- Select support surfaces to minimize PrI development.
- Discuss dressing types, descriptions, and recommendations and/or uses.
- Treatment considerations for PrI which fail to heal.

INTRODUCTION

Injuries created through pressure often manifest as a wound that must heal through secondary intention. During secondary intention, the wound is left open and heals from filling the deficit with epithelial cells and connective tissue, creating scar tissue.[1] Treatment is based on injury qualities, tailoring treatments to the characteristics of the wound and the patient's overall health status. Using principles of wound care management is foundational for all wound healing, including pressure injuries (PrI). Identifying the mechanism of injury is essential when determining care options.

Since 2008, the Centers for Medicare and Medicaid Services has considered a full-thickness PrI (stages 3, 4, and later included unstageable) that occurs while a patient is hospitalized a "preventable medical error" and would no longer pay for treatment costs associated with these injuries.[2] Prevention is ideally the best form of treatment if and when possible, and many of the basic principles are discussed in the previous journal section reviewed best practices in PrI prevention. Facility-wide policies and procedures should be developed and implemented, which include appropriate selection of therapeutic support surfaces, continued assessment of patient's nutritional status, and advanced wound care dressing selections.[3-5] Once topical intervention is deemed necessary, treatment selections should be made with interprofessional

Wound Care Team, VA Puget Sound Healthcare System, 1660 South Columbian Way, B1 R330 Seattle WA 98108, USA
* Corresponding author.
E-mail address: MelissaLHutchinsonRN@gmail.com

Crit Care Nurs Clin N Am 32 (2020) 501–520
https://doi.org/10.1016/j.cnc.2020.08.002
0899-5885/20/Published by Elsevier Inc.

ccnursing.theclinics.com

collaboration to identify products to create an environment that promotes and reduces overall healing time.

TEAM COMPOSITION

The role of an interprofessional team is to provide a diverse perspective related to direct and indirect patient care.[3] There is opportunity to implement facility-wide best practice related to pressure injury prevention (PIP) and treatment resulting in cost-effective solutions and positive outcomes. This team approach can also identify gaps in current state practice and to disseminate data specifically related to PIP or hospital-acquired pressure injury (HAPI) rates.[3,4,6]

An interprofessional plan of care should be created and discussed at least weekly with care providers.[7] This type of team approach has been shown to engage staff and contribute to culture change, which can reduce the incidence of HAPI rates.[3] Verify and coordinate so the appropriate team members are involved. Patient's family members and caregivers should be included as part of the interprofessional team because they can assist the patient with reminders to turn or reposition, can be involved in education related to ongoing treatment, or can be involved in discussions regarding goals of care.[3] The team composition may include the following:

- Providers: physician and advance practice providers
- Certified Wound Care Specialist/wound, ostomy, continence (WOC) RN
- Bedside RN and Clinical Nurse Specialist (as appropriate)
- Occupational Therapy/Physical Therapy/Speech Therapy: these colleagues may provide expert assistance on seating surfaces, movement and strength, and swallow evaluation (if needed to improve nutrition status)
- Registered Dietician: what supplements and/or micronutrients should be added to the patient's diet to optimize the healing process
- Pharmacist
- Supply chain
- Senior leadership/management
- Informatics/analytics
- Quality and safety
- Specialty ad hoc consultants (plastics, vascular, podiatry, surgery, infectious disease, dermatology)

PRESSURE INJURY TREATMENT
Basic Principles of Wound Healing

Identifying the patient's goals of care and ability to heal the wound should be accomplished by the interprofessional team as soon as possible because not all wounds have the potential for complete recovery. Factors that can impair healing in the critical care population may include comorbidities (eg, diabetes, congestive heart failure, vascular disease), severity of current illness (eg, sepsis, respiratory distress), perfusion issues (ie, peripheral vascular disease), use of vasoactive medications, and poor nutrition status.[8] A patient's intrinsic factors can affect the ability of a wound to heal and also the speed in which it may heal.

Wound healing follows a specific pattern whereby stages overlap to build and create the foundation for repair. The stages required for healing include inflammation, proliferation, angiogenesis, epidermal restoration, and wound contraction and remodeling.[1] Acute wounds following this pattern heal quickly, usually within 4 weeks. Chronic wounds do not follow this sequence and can be stuck in an unpredictable and prolonged healing pattern. As healing times prolong, it can prove challenging to treat wounds effectively. Treatment is directed at identifying the cause, supporting the host to mitigate negative healing factors, and optimizing the wound environment.[9] Choosing an appropriate advanced wound care path that provides a moist wound environment, fills dead space (when applicable), removes devitalized tissue from the wound base, and appropriately manages exudate can help to increase the potential for healing.

Appropriate wound cleansing is an important first step to preparing the wound foundation for optimal healing. Skin requires appropriate cleansing to visually assess and determine healing progression. Research supporting a particular cleansing product is inconclusive. Literature supports using either potable water or saline as equally effective in removing drainage and debris to minimize the potential for infection.[10] The presence of a wound infection can result in the impediment of wound healing, and clinical criteria may include the following[7,11]:

- Wound healing has failed to progress, or has increased in size, after 2 weeks.
- Friable tissue is apparent within the wound and bleeds easily.
- There is an increase or change in pain.
- Change in wound base color, a pale or dusky wound, may indicate poor perfusion to the wound site, impeding healing.
- Hypergranulation (red beefy wound) owing to tissue overgrowth makes it difficult for epithelial cells to migrate and appropriately fill in the wound base.
- Change in exudate amount or appearance or increase in malodorous drainage can be caused by gram-negative organisms.
- There is bridging or pocketing in the wound bed.
- There is increased erythema and/or warmth to the periwound.

Notify provider for any of the above signs and symptoms during assessment, including signs of increased white blood cells, presence of fever, tachycardia, low blood pressure, foul-smelling exudate, and/or presence of purulent drainage. Compromised patients may not demonstrate typical signs and symptoms, so a wound culture may be important in some situations if healing has stalled. If a wound culture is required, it is ideal to obtain the culture before the commencement of administering antibiotics.[12]

- Wound should be irrigated with a sterile nonantiseptic solution.
- Moisten swab of applicator with normal saline and *locate a clean area of wound base* to apply pressure, rotating the applicator 1 to 2 cm^2 over clean wound tissue.
- If a Gram stain is performed, obtain a second swab from the same site.
- Insert the swab into the appropriate sterile container, label appropriately, and transport within 1 hour to the laboratory.
- Include date, time, anatomic location of collection, and prior antibiotics administered.

Healing may also be complicated by another factor, the presence of bioburden.[12] Management of bioburden and infection topically is an adjunct to the plan of care, usually initiated by the certified wound care specialist or licensed independent practitioner (LIP) and requires regular follow-up and monitoring by the clinical consultant or provider. Clear topical instructions should be documented in the health record for the critical care nurse to follow and manage.

Basic Principles of Skin and Wound Care

Wounds heal at different rates depending on the patient's underlying condition, and wound care products can assist in the closure process. Patients with lower average mean arterial pressures (MAP) less than 75 mm Hg, low hemoglobin (<9.5 g/dL), and low albumin levels (2.8 g/dL or less) are less likely to heal than patients with higher MAPs, hemoglobin levels, and albumin levels, possibly because of tissue perfusion abnormalities, which can then disrupt healing.[13,14] Identifying factors that can enhance wound healing, while minimizing bioburden, and identifying and treating infection are critical to optimizing the local environment to encourage healing. In addition to improving the local wound environment, it is important to select advanced wound care products that can improve baseline milieu and encourage healing properties to activate even if the environment is not optimal. Advanced wound care can restore hemostasis by either donating moisture if the area is too dry or absorbing excess moisture if it is too wet. Optimizing the wound bed to create an environment that encourages epithelial growth and wound healing is the focus of advanced wound care, and product usage may change throughout the healing process as the wound bed evolves and heals.

Maintaining staff awareness and engagement is a critical part in carrying out basic principles of skin and wound care. In their study, Barakat-Johnson and colleagues[15] noted that most nurses viewed PIP as a priority, and a lack of facility PIP-related policy and clinical practice guidelines contributed to a decrease in adherence to PIP intervention.[16] Facility-wide clinical practice guidelines aid in the empowerment for the caregiver at the bedside to implement PIP and treatment related to PrI. Prevention practice, which includes offloading pressure and following a basic routine skin care regimen, should be established that enhances and protects the skin's moisture barrier and maintains the acid mantle. Microclimate can be defined as the humidity and temperature between the patient's skin and support surface. There is growing evidence in the role of microclimate in the development of stage 1 and stage 2 PrIs.[17] As humidity and temperature increases, the skin weakens and succumbs to damage related to pressure, shear, and mechanical stripping.[18] Moderately or even episodically moist skin has been associated with an increase in PrI rates in the critically ill, particularly older adults.[19] Microclimate management can be optimized through the following:

- Use of products that wick moisture away from at-risk skin
- Minimized use of layers between the patient and therapeutic support surface
- Irritants removed from the skin in a timely manner and a skin barrier applied or protectant that protects the skin from further exposure to irritants
- Control or divert the moisture source

Appropriate product selection of barrier cream or paste is part of both basic principles in skin care and the treatment plan in critically ill patients. Skin protectants should be applied directly to clean skin in a thin layer. Do not apply directly to an absorbent underpad because this can interfere with the absorptive ability of the underlying product, thus altering the microclimate. When Hoggarth and colleagues[20] studied the barrier function and skin hydration properties comparing petrolatum, dimethicone, and zinc oxide, they found zinc oxide products to provide the greatest efficacy in protecting against irritants. If urine or especially stool compromises a dressing, change the dressing to minimize risk of infection.[17] In the event stool continues to continuously compromise a silicone border multilayer prophylactic sacral dressing despite attempts to divert the source of moisture away from the dressing, consider removing the dressing and instead regularly apply a thin layer of skin protectant to the affected area in combination with offloading and microclimate management. Ensure that incontinence pads are changed frequently for incontinent patients to minimize the potential for skin breakdown related to moisture. Wet skin is more susceptible to damage; when combined with wet linen or pads, the risk of skin breakdown, injury, or infection risk almost doubles.[21]

Basic treatment of any wound should be part of the plan of care, and initial and ongoing nursing treatments and assessments should be well documented in the patient's medical record. Wound bed preparation commences with proper cleansing of the wound and periwound. All wounds, particularly those with tunneling, should be carefully cleansed and irrigated. Optimal irrigation pressure has been demonstrated to be between 4 and 15 psi, sufficient to remove debris and dressing remnants but safe for the tissue bed.[22] During irrigation, protective attire should be worn to avoid provider contamination. **Table 1** reviews cleansing agents and recommendations. Dressing selection should consider maintaining moisture balance with the exception of the presence of dry, stable eschar to the heels, which should be left intact.

Interventions and Topical Treatment Recommendations

Overlap of the PrI prevention and treatment plan of care may include the same products and interventions at times. For example, for stages 1 to 4 PrI, unstageable PrI, and deep tissue injury (DTI) located on the heel, one would still offload the injury using a pillow or heel floatation device, preventing foot drop if possible.[23,24] Multilayer silicone border foam dressings, hydrocolloids, transparent adhesives, copolymer films, and barrier creams (when applied correctly) all have the potential to cross paths as part of the PIP bundle and the topical PrI treatment plan of care. Prophylactic multilayer dressings over the heels, sacrum, under medical devices, and over any bony prominence are an adjunct and not a replacement to offloading pressure. The use of a prophylactic, silicone border multilayer foam dressing is an effective tool for managing at-risk patients (**Fig. 1**) to minimize friction and sheer. Multilayer foams enhance PIP through a variety of ways. They help to control the microclimate as they help to wick fluid and improve ventilation to the covered area. A 2015 randomized trial by Santamaria and colleagues[25] demonstrated multilayer foam dressings applied to 440 trauma or critically ill patients led to significantly fewer PrI incidents than in the control group (5 vs 20, $P = .001$). This study determined that the number needed to treat (patients using prophylactic silicone dressings) was only 10 patients receiving dressings to prevent 1 PrI. Call and colleagues[26] tested 9 commercially available dressings and observed the multilayer bordered foam's ability to reduce frictional forces and significantly reduced the presence of shear through multiple mitigating modalities. Consideration in the selection of the appropriate size dressing was noted as an important clinical decision in the preventative function of the dressing. Emerging evidence is starting to explore the lifespan of these dressings with the hopes to provide clinicians guidance in regards to dressings change frequency based on measuring the product's protective endurance as a means to enhance current best practice and potential cost-effectiveness.[27]

Dressings can serve several purposes, ranging from their efficacy for use in their role in preventing PrI in the clinical setting to serving as the primary dressing, or as secondary dressing to secure a wound filler in place in the role of treatment. An immobile patient receiving continuous renal replacement therapy with minimal ability to self-reposition may have a multilayer foam placed on the sacrum as a preventative treatment over at-risk intact skin.[25] However, in the event of an evolved PrI, the use of a multilayer foam may then transition in its use as treatment. That same multilayer silicone border foam could act as a secondary dressing over a primary dressing, such as an impregnated gauze, hydrogel, hydrofiber, calcium alginate, or collagen, in the setting of a stage 3 or stage 4 PrI. **Table 2** and **Fig. 2** provide dressing descriptions and uses. The dressing in combination with microclimate management, nutrition

256

Table 1
Cleansing agents

Agent	Description	Recommendation
Potable water	Water that is safe for drinking or cooking	• Water must be potable • No studies supporting improved wound healing over other cleansing options but adequately removes debris to provide for a clean wound base
Sterile water	Hypotonic, pH balanced between 5 and 7 pH	• No studies supporting improved wound healing over other cleansing options but adequately removes debris to provide for a clean wound base
Normal saline	Isotonic solution, often used for pressure ulcer cleansing	• Widely used in hospitals, minimal effect on reduce wound bioburden • No studies supporting improved wound healing over other cleansing options but adequately removes debris to provide for a clean wound base
Commercial agents	Ease of use due to preformulated solution (eg, Pluronic F-68 [ShurClens])	• No evidence that commercial agent (Shur-Clens) was more beneficial than normal saline or potable water
Povidone iodine	Provides antimicrobial agents for cleansing and removal of bacterial	• Cytotoxic and harmful to new tissues • May delay wound healing • May have negative systemic properties • Must be washed with normal saline or potable water after wound cleansing to minimize negative effects
Hydrogen peroxide	Antiseptic properties	• Studies demonstrate delayed wound healing • Cytotoxic and harmful to new tissues

Cleansing Practice Pearls

Minimal literature exists regarding wound healing rates and superiority of cleansing agents. The least toxic agent should be a priority with potable water and normal saline equal in the literature as cleansing options.

Wound irrigation pressure should be between 4 and 15 psi to minimize tissue trauma; a 35-mL syringe with a 19-gauge needle or 18-gauge angiocath can deliver appropriate irrigation pressure.

Abbreviations: Cath, cardiac catheterization; CRRT, continuous renal replacement therapy; IABP, intra-aortic balloon pump; SBP, systolic blood pressure; TTM, targeted temperature management.
Data from Refs.[10,12,47–49]

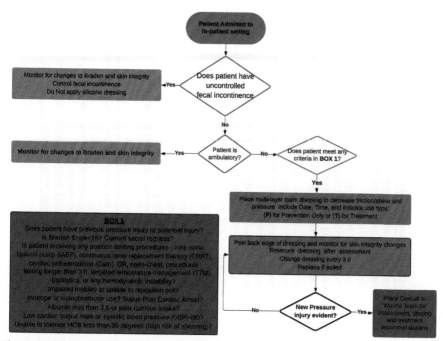

Fig. 1. Multilayer silicone dressing algorithm.

support, offloading pressure, tight glycemic control, maintaining the acid mantle of the skin, monitoring patient comfort, and patient/caregiver education may be some of the examples of the topical treatment plan that may be implemented for any stage full-thickness PrI depending on depth and exudate amount.

Dressings provide either passive or active therapy (see **Table 2**). For the purpose of this article, most dressings discussed, with the exception of negative pressure wound therapy (NPWT) and collagen, provide passive therapy. The characteristics of passive therapy include the management of exudate, protection from trauma, maintaining a moist environment, and when indicated, aid in the reduction of bacterial loads.[23,28,29]

Deep Tissue Pressure Injury

DTIs may evolve to full-thickness injuries (stage 3, 4, unstageable PrIs) and pose a challenge at the bedside for several reasons because it can be hard to determine the difference between DTI created by pressure vs cutaneous manifestations observed in the critically ill, such as ischemia, embolic showering, or other dermatologic changes associated with hemodynamic instability.[23,24,28,29] The principles of basic skin care apply with DTIs as previously discussed. In a retrospective study, contributing factors identified in the development of DTI that went on to evolve to full-thickness injury (stage 3, 4, or unstageable PrIs) included patients presenting with a diagnosis of shock, patients requiring hemodialysis, prolonged surgical procedures, and low diastolic blood pressure (poor perfusion).[30] If and when changes in the tissue are detected, ongoing intervention and assessment should be provided, as the topical plan should expect to vary as injury evolves.

Table 2
Dressing solutions

Dressing Type	Description	Comments/Recommendation
Gauze	Commonly used dressing that is moistened with saline or an antiseptic agent and can be applied to either clean or dirty wounds. Gauze comes in plain and antimicrobial forms and can be used to wick, fill, or cover a wound	• Often viewed as inexpensive, although cost of nursing time, product cost, and increased frequency of dressing change make it more costly • Nonselective, removes healthy and necrotic tissue • Potential for pain and trauma within wound bed • *When selecting gauze as a primary dressing, use a nonwoven product, moisten, and avoid overpacking the wound*
Foam	A versatile category of dressings commonly made from semiocclusive polyurethane cells and has varying capacity to absorb wound exudate. They may be impregnated or layered with antimicrobials or other materials. Also available in nonadhesive, gentle adhesive, and adhesive bordered	• Not effective in promoting autolysis • Does not donate moisture and may dehydrate granular, nondraining wounds • Can be used as a primary or a secondary dressing • Consider volume of exudate when selecting a foam dressing and frequency of dressing change
Hydrogel	Nonadherent dressings designed to donate moisture to the wound • Amorphous hydrogels are composed of water and polymers that may be impregnated to another dressing or applied directly to a wound bed • Solid gel dressings may be glycerin or water based and typically come in sheet form with or without an adhesive border	• Tends to be inexpensive • Promotes autolysis • Frequency of dressing change depends on exudate volume and type of secondary dressings • Use a moist secondary filler if needed • Use a moisture-retentive secondary dressing
Hydrofiber	Nonadherent dressings composed of sodium carboxymethylcellulose (CMC), making them highly absorptive dressings. They are available in both plain and antimicrobial forms	• Contraindicated in the setting of dry eschar, dry wound bed, third-degree burns • Indicated for use in moderate to heavy exudating wounds • Require a secondary dressing • Frequency of dressing change depends on exudate volume and type of secondary dressing used

Dressing	Description	Notes
Calcium alginate/ alginate	Nonwoven dressings composed of polysaccharide fibers or xerogel (derived from seaweed) and have the ability to absorb moderate amounts of exudate. Some alginate fibers convert to gel as they absorb exudate, resulting in an ion exchange, whereas others turn the dressing soft and moist as they absorb exudate. They are available in both plain and antimicrobial forms	• Promotes autolysis • Some alginates promote hemostasis • Irrigate the wound thoroughly following removal of an alginate from wound bed as dressing fragments may be left behind • Contraindicated in the setting of dry wound bed, or as primary dressing over tendons, joint capsules, or bone due to risk of desiccation • Frequency of dressing change depends on exudate volume and type of secondary dressing used • Provides atraumatic removal from wound bed
Transparent film/transparent adhesive	Semiocclusive/semipermeable dressings made from thin sheets of plastic with a layer of polyurethane adhesive on 1 surface. They allow moisture vapor transfer while remaining impermeable to liquids, solids, and bacteria. Transparent dressings do not have absorption capacity	• Promotes autolysis • Can be used as a primary or a secondary dressing • Waterproof • Conformability to contours of various anatomic locations • Protects from frictional injury • Allows visualization of wound
Hydrocolloid	Hydrocolloids are occlusive, made of gelatin materials, and usually come in wafer-type dressings to cover wounds. Also available in powder and paste form to fill dead space	• Should not be placed over infected wounds • Best suited for shallow, low exudating wounds • Promotes autolysis • Contraindicated in the setting of infection, fragile skin, heavy exudate • When removed, residual properties of a hydrocolloid can sometimes be mistaken for purulent exudate to an untrained caregiver/clinician • Should be changed 1-2×/wk to avoid epidermal stripping
Composite dressing	Composites are a single dressing with the components of multiple functions that contain an absorptive layer, a cover layer, and adhesive border. They may or may not be impregnated with antimicrobial agent	• Function as a primary and secondary dressing • Cover layer may be either porous or waterproof • Vary in sizes, combinations, absorptive capability • Easy to apply and relatively cost-effective

(continued on next page)

Table 2
(continued)

Dressing Type	Description	Comments/Recommendation
Copolymer dressings	Specialty absorption dressings that come in a variety of forms, such as foams, amorphous gels, liquids, and absorptive pads, with nonadherent contact layers. Copolymers bind with exudate to form a gel, resulting in a superabsorbent dressing wicking moisture from the skin. Exudate locks in the polymer resulting in the reduction of maceration of the periwound and wound bed	• May be left in place up to 7 d • May be a primary or secondary dressing • Contraindicated in the setting of dry wound bed, or as primary dressing over tendons, joint capsules, or bone due to risk of desiccation
Collagen	Usually formulated from bovine, avian, or porcine and regenerated cellulose and are considered primary dressings available in a variety of formulations. Bind to MMPs to prevent further growth factor protein degradation	• For best results apply directly to wound bed without nonviable tissue • Require a secondary dressing • Appropriate for both low and heavy exudating wounds
Negative pressure wound therapy (NPWT)	Mechanical wound care therapy that uses negative pressure to promote wound healing. Open-cell reticulated foam dressing (polyurethane or polyvinyl) fills wound base, and a seal is achieved using a semiocclusive drape, followed by application of subatmospheric pressure via tubing and mechanical computerized pump	• Dressing changes 2-3×/wk by LIP or WOC RN • Contraindicated in patients with untreated osteomyelitis, malignancy in wound, nonenteric, or unexplored fistulas, direct placement over exposed landmarks such as vessels or organs • Precautions should be taken for patients on anticoagulants or actively bleeding
Moisture barrier ointments	Petrolatum, CMC, zinc, dimethicone-based topicals that provide protection over vulnerable skin from friction and moisture	• Can be an effective topical option in hard-to-dress anatomic locations • Do not overlayer dressing to the affected area
Textile dressings	Moisture-wicking fabric designed to translocate moisture from skin folds or wounds. May come impregnated with or without antimicrobial agent	• Apply flat between skin folds • Decreases frictional injury associated with moisture • May be left in place up to 5 d or change when heavily soiled

| Enzymatic agents | Only enzyme available in the United States is collagenase, derived from Clostridium bacteria | • Selective debridement
• May be used to debride wounds with bioburden or infection
• Daily or bid application
• Wound bed must be kept moist
• Requires a secondary dressing
• Silver and cadexomer iodine inhibit or inactivate collagenase and should not be used concurrently |

Dressing Pearls

• ALL wounds including periwound skin should be cleansed with each dressing change using solutions such as normal saline, potable tap water, or commercial wound cleansers.
• When packing a wound with depth, do not overfill or overpack the wound because overpacking can contribute to trauma, interfere with perfusion, and compromise granulation tissue formation.
• When rising bacterial loads are suspected, antimicrobial topical dressings can be considered an option to provide sustained antimicrobial activity and moist wound healing.

Abbreviation: MMPs, matrix metalloproteinases.
Data from Refs.[4,41,50–52]

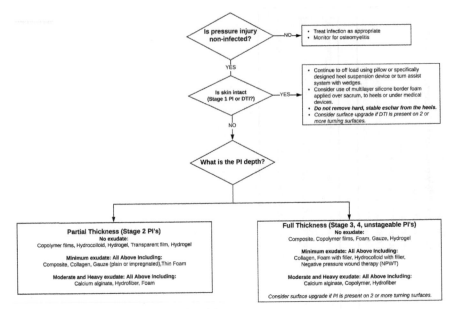

Fig. 2. Pressure injury (PrI) topicals algorithm.

Unstageable Pressure Injury

Unstageable PrI can present with adherent or loose nonviable tissue consuming all or most of the wound base. Once adequate perfusion to the wound is confirmed, consensus supports assessing for the appropriate method to remove devitalized tissue.[24] Debridement options discussed under the Dressing Selection (see **Table 2**) in this article offer options for autolytic (naturally occurring selective debridement), mechanical (nonselective), or enzymatic debridement of the wound. If sharp debridement is indicated, it should only be performed by a trained or certified specialist or LIP, and for extensive nonviable tissue, a surgical consult may be warranted. Do not debride dry, hard, nondraining eschar located on the heels; however, continue ongoing assessments every shift for changes to periwound, level of pain reported, presence of temperature change, or drainage. Utilization of a pillow or heel floatation device to offload the injury is recommended.

Upgrading the patient's therapeutic support surface may be indicated for patients who have either DTIs or unstageable PrI depending on location (trunk/pelvis). Both DTI and unstageable PrI are discussed in great depth later in the journal.

SUPPORT SURFACE SELECTION

Critical care patients are unique because of issues of immobility related to critical illness, and multiple factors can place a patient at risk for PrI development because of illness and treatment requirements. Factors that have demonstrated an effect on PrI development in critical illness include age (>70), prolonged length of stay in the intensive care unit (ICU), prolonged mechanical ventilation, number of comorbidities, severity of illness, and use of vasopressors.[31] Although patients requiring mechanical ventilation are at higher risk for PrI development, the risk has not been demonstrated to be directly related to protocols designed to reduce ventilator-associated events

(VAE). Grap and colleagues[32] determined that sacral tissue interface pressures were high in mechanically intubated patients with varying head-of-bed (HOB) elevation, although there was no correlation to an increase in PrI. Although a goal of low tissue interface pressures is optimal, additional research is needed to determine maximum tissue pressure, HOB elevation, and length of time the HOB elevation is maintained whereby friction and shearing would increase the potential for PrI development. Because many factors can influence the potential of a PrI in an Intensive Care Unit (ICU) patient, assessing the support surface function and appropriateness is important to reduce the potential for injury development. The surface should provide appropriate offloading, minimize friction and shearing, and manage microclimate effectively. Patients will have different surface needs to optimize their healing, and it is important to assess and match the patients to their appropriate surface that is available within the institution's surface selections.

Surfaces should provide optimal function within the patient's inpatient location. Critical care frame specifications are often different than a home, skilled nursing care location, or even an acute medical surgical nursing ward where advanced bedframe motions may be required (ie, lateral rotation or microclimate management). Support surfaces regarded as powered, active, or reactive surfaces that have low air loss and microclimate management features can assist in decreasing the development and progression of PrI.[33] Powered therapeutic support surfaces alter the features to immerse, envelop, and microclimate manage the patient. Air-fluidized therapy is a type of powered therapeutic support surface that forces air through a granular medium providing enhanced envelopment and immersion.[34] Therapeutic support surfaces are **not** a substitution for continuing the reposition the patient and offload pressure (**Table 3**).

If possible, avoid positioning the patient over an existing PrI. Evaluate the current surface and consider a surface upgrade for the following:

- Presence of PrI on 2 or more turning surfaces of the trunk/pelvis
- Signs of stagnation or continued deterioration of the wound despite appropriate care
- Presence of a stage 3, 4, or unstageable PrI on the trunk/pelvis
- Postflap surgery

Surfaces should allow for settings to be adjusted to the patient's weight to minimize "bottoming out," which occurs when the support surface does not elevate the patient off of the bedframe sufficiently to prevent areas of pressure. Previous approaches of performing a "hand-check" (sliding a hand between the patient the mattress to check for deflated areas) are subjective and not recommended by the National Pressure Injury Advisory Panel currently, and additional research is recommended to provide evidence-based methods of surface evaluation.[35] Assessing for any deflated cells and verifying mattress function before patient placement should be completed to minimize potential for PrI of deterioration of existing PrI. If a therapeutic support surface requires the patient's weight to be entered to calibrate zoned air cells to correctly cycle throughout the surface, confirm the patient's weigh upon admission and daily during the hospitalization to minimize the risk of injury from bottoming-out because of inappropriate weight calculations.

One additional consideration related to proper support surface function is linen and incontinence pad placement. To optimize a surface's microclimate management, and pressure redistribution capabilities, the layers between the surface and patient must be minimized. High-level evidence is currently lacking regarding the impact Safe Patient Handling and Mobility (SPHM) devices have on the integrity of the skin and the

Table 3
Therapeutic support surfaces

Surface Name	Description	Pressure Injury Most Appropriate
High-density foam (viscoelastic foam)	Reduces pressure by conforming to the patient's weight to minimize pressure areas	Stage 1 and 2 or any patient at risk for pressure injury
Low air-loss with microclimate surface	Controls temperature, humidity, and airflow to improve moisture balance near high-risk areas. Prolonged exposure to moisture can damage the skin and increase the potential for skin breakdown. A microclimate surface decreases humidity and moisture near high-risk areas decreasing the potential for skin injury development	Appropriate for all patient populations
Integrated mattress with intermittent pressure	Mattress integrated into a hospital bedframe, not an overlay or replaceable mattress. Individual cells of the mattress surface inflate and deflate intermittently to improve blood flow to high-risk areas	Appropriate for all patient populations including patients with current pressure injuries
Air-fluidized system	Self-contained electric bed/mattress system when plugged in the air pump will blow around silicone-coated beads creating a type of suspension or waterbed effect, reducing friction and shear. Also provides microclimate surface properties to control temperature, humidity, and airflow	Stage 3 and 4 pressure injury. Postmyocutaneous flap recovery or skin graft. Some wounds will become too dry in this environment; wounds should be monitored for the need of increased moisture

Support Surface Practice Pearls

Bottom or fitted linen should not be used on support surfaces; this is an additional layer, which can interfere with the beneficial low air-loss surface properties.

Minimize additional layers of incontinence pads (only use 1 pad unless severe diarrhea is present, then frequent cleansing and pad change are necessary).

Float heels to reduce potential for heel ulcers: Offload heels with a commercial device or with pillows placed beneath calves, suspending the heels off the edge of pillow to completely relieve heel pressure. Knees should be slightly bent to minimize pressure on the Achilles tendon and obstruction of the popliteal vein. Floating heels does not prevent plantar flexion contracture or drop foot; for nonresponsive patients, a commercial device that can decrease heel pressure and protect plantar flexion contracture is advised.

Verify surface function prior to patient placement.

Data from Serraes B, van Leen M, Schols J, et al. Prevention of pressure ulcers with a static air support surface: A systematic review. Int Wound J. 2018;15(3):333–43.

potential for altering microclimate and/or contributing the development of PrI.[36] Check SPHM devices for appropriateness, which includes verifying they are made from an appropriate material that can be left under the patient because this counts as a layer between the patient and therapeutic support surface. The more layers present, the less airflow will reach the patient, making it more difficult to regulate the patient's temperature and moisture level. Limit the layers between the patient and use incontinence and repositioning devices that are appropriate for the surface. Fitted sheets should properly fit over mattresses and integrated therapeutic support surfaces and should be avoided over low air loss mattress replacement systems because of the potential for hammocking, compromising the therapeutic effect of the surface. Do not place a fitted sheet over air-fluidized therapy.

Treatment Considerations

Osteomyelitis

Osteomyelitis can be a challenge to diagnose; it is defined as a bone infection characterized by a mixture of inflammatory cells, bone necrosis, and new bone formation resulting as a complication from a wound infection.[12] Osteomyelitis can be characterized as acute (occurs for <6 weeks after initially diagnosed) or chronic (lasts longer than 6 weeks and symptoms return). Notify the provider for clinical assessment that includes visualization of exposed bone, worsening wound, or wound that persists for greater than 1 month. In diabetic patients with PrI to the lower extremities or heels, a thorough history, including prior amputation, renal insufficiency, and recurrent foot ulcer, should also be obtained to aid in diagnosis identification. Consider obtaining laboratory values, such as complete blood count because elevated white blood cell counts may be present as well as erythrocyte sedimentation rate and C-reactive protein. The presence of osteomyelitis is best confirmed by obtaining a bone biopsy, which is not always feasible in the critical care population because this requires the patient be sent to the operating room to obtain the biopsy sample. Diagnostic imaging includes MRI, and in foot wounds that probe-to-bone a plain radiography can confirm or exclude diagnosis.[37,38]

When osteomyelitis is suspected or confirmed, use of a topical antimicrobial dressing or irrigation solution can be considered as an adjunct to supporting the basic principles of wound healing and topical management in collaboration with an infectious disease provider and the interprofessional team. It is imperative to maintain continued surveillance of the patient's nutritional status and comorbidities and to reduce immunosuppressive therapies if appropriate.[38] Surgical consultation should be considered in cases whereby there is concern of advancing cellulitis or sepsis, a stage 3 or 4 PrI that is not closing despite comprehensive treatment, or if an unstageable PrI requires further debridement because of the presence of extensive necrotic tissue.[39]

Tissue flaps

Surgical tissue flaps are commonly used to treat PrI and involve the reconstruction of underlying structures to fill a deficit. After a flap surgery, the patient will be placed on an upgraded therapeutic support surface, such as air-fluidized therapy or low air loss surface. Flap protocols should be used to assess the vascular status of the flap: Signs of flap necrosis present as areas of cool or cold skin that may appear blue, purple, or black. It is important to reduce shear and friction on the surgical site and avoid pulling or dragging of the patient during repositioning. A flap protocol can provide practice guidance to minimize complications, including dehiscence or failure of wound healing, which can lead to additional procedures. Asanza and colleagues[40] studied flap protocols, specifically whether 6 weeks versus 4 weeks of postoperative bedrest protocols decreased complications. No significant difference in 6 weeks of bedrest versus 4 weeks was identified; because of the increase in hospital costs, potential for hospital-associated infections, and impact on quality of life, an additional 2 weeks of bedrest is not warranted. Outcomes from this study demonstrated the importance of a standard flap protocol with interprofessional team collaboration.

Negative pressure wound therapy

NPWT is a relatively safe modality that uses subatmospheric pressure through the act of suction to facilitate wound healing, indicated for acute and chronic wounds, and may be considered as an early adjunct therapy for stage 3 and 4 PrI.[24,41] A certified wound care specialist or LIP will assess the wound and patient's condition for appropriateness of initiation of NPWT and will usually be responsible for managing the routine dressing changes. Tubing that is connected to the NPWT dressing should be positioned in a way to minimize or avoid pressure. Repositioning critically ill patients with tubes and lines frequently pose increased risk for the development of medical device-related PrI. Close monitoring is indicated in patient populations at high risk for bleeding or in patients presenting with sepsis or with local infection because the application of NPWT is contraindicated in the setting of untreated osteomyelitis. Do not remove the NPWT dressing unless instructed by the certified wound care specialist or LIP, and notify the provider if therapy loses its seal or therapy is turned off for greater than 2 hours.[42] Ongoing documentation should include quantity and consistency of the output from the wound in the NPWT pump's canister, integrity of the dressing's seal, confirmation of pump's settings, intervention provided (eg, canister change, troubleshooting dressing seal), and patient's tolerance to therapy each shift.

Palliative care

Approximately 1 in 5 deaths occur in or shortly after an ICU admission, which regularly is faced with the challenges of addressing and readdressing goals of care.[43,44] Transition to palliative wound care may be required when prior comprehensive interventions have become futile and end of life is imminent. The topical goal of care for treating palliative PrI is prioritized pain control, quality of life, and providing patient dignity. These goals can be achieved by appropriate management of exudate, odor, and the prevention of bleeding or trauma.[45] Topical dressing selection should appropriately manage exudate, minimize contamination of the wound resulting in the need for increased frequency of dressing changes, close monitoring for adequate pain management systemically and topically if needed. Topical metronidazole may be considered for use in wounds where odor is present, particularly in the presence of anaerobic bacteria. In nonverbal patients, agitation, increased respiration, or grimacing may be signs the patient is poorly tolerating topical intervention. There may be case-by-case scenarios where NPWT is indicated in the topical management of PrI during end of life, and these scenarios require continued assessment by the certified wound care specialist or LIP.

SUMMARY

Even with the most rigorous prevention methods, PrI may still develop among compromised patients. The development of a PrI may lead to costly treatments, may lead to an increase in patient's hospital length of stay, and can contribute to a patient's deterioration and even death. Use of appropriate support surfaces, adequate offloading, and advanced wound care products are critical to optimize healing and prevent further deterioration of a PrI.[46]

A variety of advanced wound care options could be appropriate for a patient, depending on their comorbidities, critical illness, and ability to heal. The best treatment approaches are ones that provide a moist wound environment, fill dead space, and remove devitalized tissue. An interprofessional team can collaborate to create the most appropriate treatment plan using advanced wound care products and comprehensive care planning. Even with optimal treatments, some wounds will fail to heal and require more invasive methods, including surgical interventions. Not every treatment will work for every patient, so tailoring the treatment with the interprofessional teams' input will benefit the patient and potentially decrease the number of days required to treat a PrI.

DISCLOSURE

The authors have nothing to disclose.

REFERENCES

1. Doughty D, Sparks B. Wound-healing physiology and factors that affect the repair process. In: Bryant R, Nix D, editors. Acute and chronic wounds: current management concepts. St. Louis (MO): Elsevier; 2016. p. 63–81.
2. Kuhn H. State Medicaid director letter. In: Kuhn HB, editor. Memorandum SMDL #08-004, Center for Medicaid and State Operations. Baltimore (MD): 2008. p. 5. Available at: https://downloads.cms.gov/cmsgov/archived-downloads/SMDL/downloads/SMD073108.pdf. Accessed January 11, 2020.
3. Miller MW, Emeny RT, Freed GL. Reduction of hospital-acquired pressure injuries using a multidisciplinary team approach: a descriptive study. Wounds 2019; 31(4):108–13.
4. Black J, Fletcher J, Harding K, et al. Role of dressings in pressure ulcer prevention 2016.
5. Vargo D, Bryant R. Billing, reimbursement, and setting up a clinic. In: Bryant R, Nix D, editors. Acute and chronic wounds: current management concepts. 5th edition. St. Louis (MO): Elsevier; 2016. p. 21–39.
6. Ahroni JH. Developing a wound and skin care program. J Wound Ostomy Continence Nurs 2014;41(6):549–55.
7. Sibbald RG, Goodman L, Woo KY, et al. Special considerations in wound bed preparation 2011: an update©. Adv Skin Wound Care 2011;24(9):415–36 [quiz: 37–8].
8. Leaper D, Assadian O, Edmiston CE. Approach to chronic wound infections. Br J Dermatol 2015;173(2):351–8.
9. Rolstad B, Ermer-Seltun J. Module I: principles of wound management, topical therapy: WebWoc nursing education program. 2019. p. 8, 16, 17, 18, 19.
10. Resende MM, Rocha CA, Correa NF, et al. Tap water versus sterile saline solution in the colonisation of skin wounds. Int Wound J 2016;13(4):526–30.
11. Gould L, Stuntz M, Giovannelli M, et al. Wound Healing Society 2015 Update on Guidelines for pressure ulcers. Wound Repair Regen 2016;24(1):145–62.
12. Stotts N. Wound infection: diagnosis and management. In: Bryant R, Nix D, editors. Acute and chronic wounds: current management concepts. St. Louis (MO): Elsevier; 2016. p. 283–94.
13. Karahan A, AAbbasoğlu A, Isik SA, et al. Factors affecting wound healing in individuals with pressure ulcers: a retrospective study. Ostomy Wound Manage 2018;64(2):32–9.

14. Sung YH, Park KH. Factors affecting the healing of pressure ulcers in a Korean acute care hospital. J Wound Ostomy Continence Nurs 2011;38(1):38–45.

15. Barakat-Johnson M, Barnett C, Wand T, et al. Knowledge and attitudes of nurses toward pressure injury prevention: a cross-sectional multisite study. J Wound Ostomy Continence Nurs 2018;45(3):233–7.

16. Dilie A, Mengistu D. Assessment of nurses', knowledge, attitude, and perceived barriers to expressed pressure ulcer prevention practice in Addis Ababa Government hospitals, Addis Ababa, Ethiopia, 2015. Adv Nurs 2015;2015:11.

17. Kottner J, Cuddigan J, Carville K, et al. Prevention and treatment of pressure ulcers/injuries: the protocol for the second update of the international Clinical Practice Guideline 2019. J Tissue Viability 2019;28(2):51–8.

18. Gray M, Black JM, Baharestani MM, et al. Moisture-associated skin damage: overview and pathophysiology. J Wound Ostomy Continence Nurs 2011;38(3): 233–41.

19. Alderden J, Cummins MR, Pepper GA, et al. Midrange Braden subscale scores are associated with increased risk for pressure injury development among critical care patients. J Wound Ostomy Continence Nurs 2017;44(5):420–8.

20. Hoggarth A, Waring M, Alexander J, et al. A controlled, three-part trial to investigate the barrier function and skin hydration properties of six skin protectants. Ostomy Wound Manage 2005;51(12):30–42.

21. Gerhardt LC, Strassle V, Lenz A, et al. Influence of epidermal hydration on the friction of human skin against textiles. J R Soc Interface 2008;5(28):1317–28.

22. Whitney J, Phillips L, Aslam R, et al. Guidelines for the treatment of pressure ulcers. Wound Repair Regen 2006;14(6):663–79.

23. Wound, Ostomy and Continence Nurses Society-Wound Guidelines Task Force. WOCN 2016 guideline for prevention and management of pressure injuries (ulcers): an executive summary. J Wound Ostomy Continence Nurs 2017;44(3): 241–6.

24. Haesler E. Prevention and treatment of pressure ulcers/injuries: quick reference guide. In: European Pressure Ulcer Advisory Panel NPIAPaPPPIA, editor. Australia: Cambridge Media; 2019.

25. Santamaria N, Gerdtz M, Sage S, et al. A randomised controlled trial of the effectiveness of soft silicone multi-layered foam dressings in the prevention of sacral and heel pressure ulcers in trauma and critically ill patients: the Border Trial. Int Wound J 2015;12(3):302–8.

26. Call E, Pedersen J, Bill B, et al. Enhancing pressure ulcer prevention using wound dressings: what are the modes of action? Int Wound J 2015;12(4):408–13.

27. Burton JN, Fredrickson AG, Capunay C, et al. New clinically relevant method to evaluate the life span of prophylactic sacral dressings. Adv Skin Wound Care 2019;32(7S Suppl 1):S14–20.

28. Edsberg LE, Black JM, Goldberg M, et al. Revised national pressure ulcer advisory panel pressure injury staging system: revised pressure injury staging system. J Wound Ostomy Continence Nurs 2016;43(6):585–97.

29. Lachenbruch C, Ribble D, Emmons K, et al. Pressure ulcer risk in the incontinent patient: analysis of incontinence and hospital-acquired pressure ulcers from the international pressure ulcer Prevalence™ survey. J Wound Ostomy Continence Nurs 2016;43(3):235–41.

30. Kirkland-Kyhn H, Teleten O, Wilson M. A retrospective, descriptive, comparative study to identify patient variables that contribute to the development of deep tissue injury among patients in intensive care units. Ostomy Wound Manage 2017; 63(2):42–7.

31. Cox J. Pressure injury risk factors in adult critical care patients: a review of the literature. Ostomy Wound Manage 2017;63(11):30–43.

32. Grap MJ, Munro CL, Schubert CM, et al. Lack of association of high backrest with sacral tissue changes in adults receiving mechanical ventilation. Am J Crit Care 2018;27(2):104–13.

33. Black J, Berke C, Urzendowski G. Pressure ulcer incidence and progression in critically ill subjects: influence of low air loss mattress versus a powered air pressure redistribution mattress. J Wound Ostomy Continence Nurs 2012;39(3): 267–73.

34. Panel NPIA. Terms and definitions related to support surfaces. Support surface standards initiative. Westford, MA: 2019.

35. Call E, Deppisch M, Jordan R, et al. Hand check method: is it an effective method to monitor for bottoming out?. In: A national pressure ulcer advisory position statement. Westford, MA: National Pressure Ulcer Advisory Panel; 2015.

36. Brienza D, Deppisch M, Gillespie C, et al. Do lift slings significantly change the efficacy of therapeutic support surfaces?. In: A national pressure ulcer advisory panel white paper. Westford, MA: National Pressure Ulcer Advisory Panel; 2015.

37. Weir D, Schultz G. Assessment and management of wound-related infections. In: Doughty D, McNichol L, editors. Wound, Ostomy and Continence Nurses Society® core curriculum: wound management. Philadelphia: Wolters Kluwer Health; 2015. p. 168–9.

38. European Pressure Ulcer Advisory Panel NPUAP, and Pan Pacific Pressure Injury Alliance. Infection and Biofilms. Prevention and treatment of pressure ulcers/injuries: methodology protocol for the clinical practice guideline. 3rd edition. Westford, MA: EPUAP, NPUAP, PPPIA; 2019. p. 251–66.

39. European Pressure Ulcer Advisory Panel NPUAP, and Pan Pacific Pressure Injury Alliance. Cleansing and debridement prevention and treatment of pressure ulcers/injuries: methodology protocol for the clinical practice guideline. 3rd edition. Westford, MA: EPUAP, NPUAP, PPPIA; 2019. p. 237–50.

40. Asanza JL, Matsuwaka ST, Keys K, et al. Comparing 4- and 6-week post-flap protocols in patients with spinal cord injury. J Spinal Cord Med 2019;1–7. https://doi.org/10.1080/10790268.2019.1703501.

41. Netsch D, Nix D, Haugen V. Negative pressure wound therapy. In: Bryant R, Nix D, editors. Acute and chronic wounds: current management concepts. St. Louis (MO): Elsevier; 2016. p. 350–60.

42. KCI. V.A.C therapy, clinical guidelines a reference source for clinicians. KCI Licensing, Inc; 2014.

43. Swetz KM, Mansel JK. Ethical issues and palliative care in the cardiovascular intensive care unit. Cardiol Clin 2013;31(4):657–68.

44. Chow K. Ethical dilemmas in the intensive care unit: treating pain and symptoms in noncommunicative patients at the end of life. J Hosp Palliat Nurs 2014;16(5): 256–60.

45. Walsh AF, Bradley M, Cavallito K. Management of fungating tumors and pressure ulcers in a patient with stage IV cutaneous malignant melanoma. J Hosp Palliat Nurs 2014;16(4):208–14.

46. Padula WV, Delarmente BA. The national cost of hospital-acquired pressure injuries in the United States. Int Wound J 2019;16(3):634–40.

47. Wilkins RG, Unverdorben M. Wound cleaning and wound healing: a concise review. Adv Skin Wound Care 2013;26(4):160–3.

48. Sibbald RG, Elliott JA, Verma L, et al. Update: topical antimicrobial agents for chronic wounds. Adv Skin Wound Care 2017;30(10):438–50.

49. Fernandez R, Griffiths R, Ussia C. Effectiveness of solutions, techniques and pressure in wound cleansing. JBI Libr Syst Rev 2004;2(7):1–55.

50. Jaszarowski K, Murphree R. Wound cleansing and dressing selection. In: Doughty D, McNichol L, editors. Wound, Ostomy and Continence Nurses Society® core curriculum: wound management. Philadelphia: Wolters Kluwer Health; 2015. p. 131–44.

51. Ramundo J. Wound debridement. In: Bryant R, Nix D, editors. Acute and chronic wounds: current management concepts. St. Louis (MO): Elsevier; 2016. p. 295–305.

52. Bryant R, Nix D. Principles of wound healing and topical management. In: Bryant R, Nix D, editors. Acute and chronic wounds: current management concepts. St. Louis (MO): Elsevier; 2016. p. 306–24.

Pressure Injury Prevention and Treatment in Critically Ill Children

Ann Marie Nie, RN, MSN, APRN, FNP-BC, CWOCN

KEYWORDS

- Pressure injury • Ulcer • Children • Neonates • NICU • CVICU • PICU

KEY POINTS

- Pediatric pressure injury prevention is a multidisciplinary responsibility.
- Developmental differences in anatomy and physiology inform pressure injury risk in the pediatric patient.
- Repositioning hemodynamically unstable pediatric patients should be undertaken using a slow, incremental approach.
- Products that have known safety in children are amorphous hydrogels, honey dressings, polyhexamethylene biguanide, collagen, 3% bismuth tribromophenate, and petrolatum.

INTRODUCTION

Prevention of pediatric pressure injuries (PI) has historically looked to adult prevention measures to guide practice. The conundrum for PI prevention is that many of the adult prevention measures may not apply to the developing child (eg, applying foam dressing over the coccyx, or use of barrier creams/ointments to decrease moisture related to PI development over the sacrum when the child is not toilet trained).[1]

The National Pressure Injury Advisory Panel released an updated White Paper in 2019, "Pressure Injuries in the Pediatric Population: A National Pressure Ulcer Advisory Panel White Paper."[2] The paper notes PI incidence is highest in the pediatric critical care areas, up to 43.1%, underscoring the importance of PI prevention in that population.

The White Paper recommends organizing PI prevention efforts by the age of the developing child. This suggestion is related to the anatomy and physiology of the developing skin of the child. Depending upon the age of the neonate at birth, the stratum corneum is thinner and may only be 2 to 3 cell layers,[3] whereas a full-term infant has 10 to 20 layers.[3–5] Neonates younger than 24-weeks' gestation may have no stratum corneum.[3] This lack of stratum corneum makes it difficult to stage a PI in this very young population accurately. Neonates born less than 32 weeks' gestation tend to

National Pressure Injury Advisory Panel, Children's Minnesota Hospital and Clinics, 2525 Chicago Avenue, Minneapolis, MN 55404, USA
E-mail addresses: annmarie.nie@childrensmn.org; annmarienie@gmail.com

Crit Care Nurs Clin N Am 32 (2020) 521–531
https://doi.org/10.1016/j.cnc.2020.08.003
0899-5885/20/© 2020 Elsevier Inc. All rights reserved.

have dry and scaly skin related to the immature properties of the skin for protection and absorption.[5] They will be placed in a high-humidity environment to assist in maturing the skin. The increased humidity is a contributing moisture factor under medical devices for PI development.

Age is an important consideration in terms of tissue distribution relative to PI risk. For example, as the child ages, the occipital becomes more of a concern for PI development. The occipital in infants and up to age 5 is proportionally larger than their body and will absorb the weight against a surface if not protected.[6] Children's feet have an increase in adipose tissue relative to adults, and the cartilage of their skeletal system weighs less, potentially resulting in a decrease risk for heel PIs.

This article describes best practice in PI prevention among pediatric critical care patients, with attention to unique age-related considerations. Best practices in the areas of neonatal intensive care unit (NICU), cardiovascular intensive care unit (CVICU), and pediatric intensive care unit (PICU) are described.

BACKGROUND

There are 3 primary types of PICUs. The PICU provides care for critically ill infants, children, and young adults up to age 21. The CVICU treats patients from infancy to adulthood with life-threatening congenital heart disease. The NICU treats premature neonates and infants as young as 23 weeks' gestation.

PREVENTION INTERVENTIONS
Skin and Tissue Assessment

Skin assessment is a standard for PI prevention.[1] Clinical guidelines suggest that a skin assessment should be performed on admission (to the facility and unit), as part of a standard risk assessment, and with any change in condition that may increase the patient's risk of PI development, and before discharge.[1] Abnormal skin concerns should be documented in the medical record.

Preventive Skin Care

Pediatric hospitals may limit the products that are available for use in skin maintenance to products that can be used on all patients. The skin of the neonate does not have a well-developed barrier function and will absorb certain products causing skin damage.[3] To prevent central line-associated bloodstream infection, Solutions for Patient Safety[7,8] recommends daily chlorhexidine gluconate (CHG) baths for children older than 2 months of age with a central venous catheter. CHG may cause dry skin.[9] It is imperative to apply moisturizer after the bath. The moisturizer needs to be compatible with CHG to avoid removing the prevention from infection that CHG provides. It is recommended to apply a silicone moisturizer, such a dimethicone.[5]

Normal cleansing of the skin in the NICU is performed with water wipes or normal saline. Dimethicone moisturizer can be used in children of all ages for dryness and to promote barrier function. It is acceptable to add mild soap for bathing infants greater than 2 months of age.[10] As the child enters puberty, it is important to bath the patient with mild soap and water along with the CHG bath. There should be minimally 1 hour between the 2 baths not to diminish the effectiveness of CHG.[11]

Continence Management

In adults, sacrococcygeal PI development is associated with incontinence.[1] However, children less than 3 years of age are incontinent related to their development.[12] Both fecal incontinence and urinary incontinence are associated with diaper dermatitis in children.[13] Currently research is absent to correlate incontinence with PI development in developmental normal incontinent children under the age of 3. Clinicians and caregivers are aware of the association with dermatitis and adopt a frequent changing schedule.[10] Barrier creams are encouraged for any child in diapers.

Expert opinion connects PI development in older children (school-age to young adult) with immobility and neurologic conditions, ie, myelomeningocele.[1] Children with these conditions do not have bowel and bladder continence. The sensation for movement and moisture is either decreased or absent, and the combination of immobility and moisture is a known risk factor for PI development.[1] It is important in this population to develop a bowel and bladder program, along with a mobility schedule.

Nutrition

A standard does not exist for PI prevention related to nutrition in the pediatric population. All nutritional guidelines are related to growth and development, or malnutrition. It is important for the interdisciplinary care team to include dieticians who are aware of how nutritional requirements impact PI development and healing. Seattle Children's has developed a pathway to optimize nutrition for wound healing.[14] This pathway does not focus on prevention, but on healing once the wound is present. Nutritional screening should include energy expenditures, edema, and fluid shifts.

Repositioning and Early Mobilization

PI develop because of increased pressure on soft tissues. If the pressure is removed, a PI is unable to form. This principle is at the forefront of prevention. Individuals normally move positions when the discomfort of pressure is felt. Pediatric patients less than 5 years old have difficulty differentiating sensation. Hunger pains can elicit the same response as pain. They may state that something hurts when the sensation is either a cooling sensation or one of burning. Infants are unable to tell the caregiver that there is discomfort except for crying. A child in the intensive care unit (ICU) may be sedated for medical reasons and therefore unable to communicate discomfort. The bedside clinician has the responsibility to move the patient when the patient is unable to perform this prevention measure.

Quality improvement studies have been performed to determine whether the standard every 2-hour repositioning is appropriate for the pediatric hospitalized patient.[15,16] Randomized controlled trials have not been performed related to timing of repositioning of the pediatric patient. The generally accepted practice is to adopt the adult timing of q 2 hours, excluding the NICU.[1]

Repositioning in the Neonatal Intensive Care Unit

In the NICU, a full skin assessment and re-positioning should be performed during cares. The neonate is in the process of normal fetal central nervous system development. It is important that the NICU has instituted neuroprotective interventions. One strategy for neurodevelopment is sleep and decreasing of external stimulus. Adequate rest and sleep may be the single most important strategy for the preterm infant's long-term neurologic success.[17] For these reasons, the neonate is typically not disturbed except for cares every 4 hours. Surfaces are used to assist with off-loading; these are discussed under support surfaces.

Repositioning in the Cardiovascular Intensive Care Unit and Pediatric Intensive Care Unit

In the cardiac population, importance is placed on oxygenation. The heart condition may cause decreased perfusion to the extremities and predispose the skin to ischemic episodes. In the author's clinical practice, these ischemic skin conditions can mimic deep tissue PI. Patients in cardiac failure may require life saving devices such as extracorporeal membrane oxygenation (ECMO) and ventricular assist devices for their medical condition. These lifesaving equipment exert external pressure to the skin at the cannulation sites. As healthcare makes advances in life saving measures, heart failure patients have an increase in susceptibility to skin complications. As medicine becomes more adept at lifesaving measures, heart failure patients may have skin complications. Documentation of PI prevention measures is important to determine if a PI that develops was preventable. If prevention measures were not documented, it would be unclear if the PI could have been prevented.

Typically, the CVICU and PICU have adopted the adult standard of repositioning the patient every 2 hours. The hemodynamically unstable patient requires a slow repositioning approach. Repositioning requires 2 – 3 staff members depending on the size of the child. One for the head and shoulders, one for the back and abdomen and one for the legs. If the child is smaller, two individuals can perform: one for the head and back and one for the abdomen and legs. The movement should be coordinated. As the patient is moved from the supine position to a tilt, any signs of a decrease in blood pressure or pulse should halt the movement in the tilt. The patient should not be returned to the supine position. Wait for the vitals to stabilize and complete the turn. Check to make sure that the coccyx can be felt and is adequately positioned off of the surface. Positioning devices should be applied to the child to maintain the change in position. Prior to repositioning, adequately pre-medicate the patient for pain control.

Repositioning a patient in bed is aimed at relieving pressure over bony prominences, particularly the occiput, sacrococcygeal region, and heels. Children in different stages of development are also in different stages of bone ossification. The neonate's skeleton initiates as a cartilaginous scaffold. This continues until puberty when hormones initiate the process of ossification, and endochondral bone is formed and the growth plates are fused.[18] Because of this process of normal development, the skeletal structure of children who have not yet reached puberty do not have the weight of fully formed bones. Without the same weight to the skeletal system as an adult, it is unknown if neonates to school-aged children require the same diligence of offloading the heels and sacrococcygeal area as is required in adults.

Occipital Repositioning

Neonates and infants

The weight of the skull in neonates and infants rests on the occipital ridge. Close attention to this this body part is required for PI prevention. As the patient is repositioned, the head should also be turned following the body (ie, if the patient is repositioned to the left side, the head should be positioned to the left, offloading the posterior aspect). Patients on ECMO support require attention to the cannulas when repositioning. Cannulation is typically performed in the right jugular. The cannulas are sutures to the right neck and scalp. This site is protected during movement. The use of a fluidized positioned assists in stabilization of the head during movement and supports the cannulas.

The scalp of patients with vEEG leads should be protected from MDRPI. Patients lying directly on a surface will have pressure from the leads. To assist in offloading, a fluidized positioning or polyurethane foam can be applied. The leads "sink" into the product and do not exert pressure against the scalp.

Children 5 years and older have the weight of the head further up on the skull.[6] It is located just above the occipital ridge. The same principle applies when repositioning; the head follows the turn. The head should not be left in a midline position as the body is turned.

Sacrococcygeal Repositioning

Neonates, infants, and toddler

Research is lacking to determine if this population has an increased propensity for PI over the sacrococcygeal region. Without the evidence, we continue to follow the recommendation for adults. Adult studies suggest repositioning should be conducted at a 30° angle.[1] Evidence for an ideal turn angle in the pediatric population is lacking. Children have a much smaller width, and 30° can position them on their trochanter. Lacking evidence, it becomes important for the clinician performing the repositioning to palpate the coccyx to determine that it is not being used as a pivot point and has been adequately offloaded.

School age and older

As this age group enters puberty, the standard continues to be offloading the coccyx and not allowing it to be a pivot point. Adolescents and young adults should follow the adult standard of 30° angle as their body proportions mimic an adult's.

Positioning for Ventilator-Associated Pneumonia and Pressure Injury Prevention

Ventilator-associated pneumonia has bundle elements that consist of elevating the head of the bed 30° to 45°. To prevent sliding and shearing, clinicians will apply a rolled blanket, a pillow, or a fluidized positioner under the thighs. This position puts children in a "V" position with the weight of their body on the occiput and the coccyx. The V position should be avoided. It is best practice to apply a fluidized positioner to the calves, elevating the heels off the bed and preventing sliding. This position allows for the body weight to be distributed over the sacrococcygeal region and buttocks, thus decreasing the potential of a PI. The posterior scalp should be offloaded in the reclining position. Fluidized positioners and gel pillows have anecdotally been used to successfully offload the scalp.

Prophylactic Dressings to the Sacrococcygeal Region

There is a lack of evidence to show that prophylactic dressings are an effective intervention in the pediatric population. Anecdotally, individual pediatric hospitals have reporting instituting application of foam dressings for critically ill patients or those with surgeries lasting greater than 3 hours. Consensus does not exist as to the pediatric age range that will benefit from the application of the dressing. Best practice is to reposition the patient every 2 hours, thereby relieving the pressure to the sacrococcygeal skin. A foam dressing application should not take the place of repositioning a patient.

Repositioning Heels

Neonates, infants, and toddlers

As discussed earlier, it is unknown if neonates, infants, and toddlers have enough weight to their heels to cause PI. Their feet have more adipose tissue than adults, and the cartilage of the skeletal system is not as heavy. Best practice is to continue to elevate for comfort until research is performed.

School-age, teenagers, and young adults

Puberty in boys starts between ages 12 and 16 and will last through age 21; in girls, puberty starts between ages 9 and 14 and lasts through age 18. During puberty, the skeletal structure undergoes ossification and weight increases in the heels as the adipose tissue decreases. This changes creates greater concern for PI development in the heels. Research is unavailable to determine the appropriate age when offloading the heels becomes a necessary component for PI prevention. Best practice remains to elevate the heels off the surface. Adult studies show that a prophylactic dressing may be effective in assisting in prevention.[1] It is best, Appropriate elevation requires that the caregiver's hand will slide under the heel without touching the foot.

Support Surfaces

Premature hospitalized patients present unique challenges. The patient is medically fragile and needs to be given the opportunity to develop as normally as possible. For developmental reasons, it is best to put the patient in a position that mimics the mother's womb. NICUs do this by using devices that help to create a "nesting" environment. Blanket rolls and positioning aids are used to mold around the patient to create a barrier environment. Fluidized positioners can also be used to create a 'nest. Infants and neonates are positioned on positioner and the sides are molded upward to create the "nest." This nest assists with neurodevelopment[19] by facilitating increased sleep. The fluidized positioner also offloads the occiput to assist in PI prevention. The positioner is made of medical-grade oil and air in a polyurethane covering. The patient should not be positioned directly on the positioner but should have 1 layer between the patient and the positioner. A full-body positioner can be used for neonates and infants until they reach a stage of movement, and the positioner is too restrictive. Then, the positioner should be removed and the patient put in a crib.[20]

CVICUs and PICUs typically use full-size beds for staff convenience when the patient is critically ill and sedated. The open bed allows for easy access to the patient for procedures and is not as restrictive as a crib. The American Academy of Pediatrics issued updates related to safe sleep for infants[21] that discourages the use of memory foam as a surface. This surface conforms to the weight of the body and poses a risk of suffocation for children unable to shift their weight and move their head independently. Manufacturers of full air mattresses recommend that they not be used on patient's weighing less than 70 lbs. These limitations can create a unique set of concerns in purchasing pressure redistribution surfaces for the population. One study suggests that a foam overlay provides PI relief in pediatrics.[22] Overlays are an additional cost to the facility but prevention of PI may outweigh the additional cost. Bed manufacturers may work with pediatric hospitals to create surfaces that can accommodate the unique needs of this population. Air surfaces should be reserved for teenagers and young adults with needs that cannot be addressed on a foam surface.

Positioning Devices

A fluidized positioner, as described above, can be used as a surface for neonates and infants. This same positioner can be used for positioning support in any age child. The moldability of the positioner allows it to be shaped into the contours of the patient allowing for offloading of bony prominences.

Pediatric hospitals also use "bendy shapers" to mold under the legs of the patient and up the sides to create containment. These bendy shapers are soft and washable. Rolled blankets are also used to extend the neck of patients with tracheostomies and to the midback for chest expansion of patients in the CVICU. It is the opinion of this author that blanket rolls should be discouraged. Blanket rolls have caused stage 3 PI to the neck and midback when used for an extended time in this author's clinical practice. A blanket roll exerts increased pressure on the soft tissue and does not allow for offloading of pressure. Application of blanket rolls under a patient should be used with caution.

Pillows continue to be used for positioning and are readily available. Expert opinion suggests that pillows can be used for elevating of heels, but should be used with caution on the occipital in a sedated patient because they do not have offloading capabilities.[1]

Medical Device-Related Pressure Injury

Medical devices are the leading cause of PI in pediatrics.[2] Lifesaving care cannot be instituted without the use of these devices. As such, pediatric hospitals should institute a plan for prevention related to medical devices while continuing to provide care to the ICU patient. **Table 1** outlines a suggested plan for preventing medical decide–related pressure injures.

TREATMENT

Wounds in pediatrics follow the same trajectory as in adults; however, fibroblasts, collagen, and elastin occur in greater numbers, and granulation tissue forms faster than in adults.[23] The expectation by many providers is that the wound will heal with little interference. However, wounds will stall in pediatrics just as in adults.[23] Intervention is a necessary component of wound healing.

Cleansing

Wounds with disrupted skin should be cleansed using aseptic technique. This requires a solution and preferably gauze to remove any tissue fragments and products in the wound the impede healing. Solutions can be normal saline or a wound cleanser that does not disturb the fibroblasts and is safe for neonates.[23]

Debridement

All ages of children can develop slough and eschar in a wound bed. In the NICU, the author has experienced premature infants typically healing the wound covered with eschar without intervention. It is best to take a watch-and-wait approach in this population. The eschar lifts off leaving new epithelium. If any signs or symptoms of infection are noted, the wound should be gently derided using autolytic debridement. This can be accomplished by application of amorphous hydrogel or a honey dressing to the wound bed with a foam outer dressing.[23] Dressing should be changed 3 to 2 times weekly.

PI with necrosis in school-age and older patients without a cardiac diagnosis should be debrided. The slough and eschar will impede healing.[23–25] All methods used in adults can also be used in this population: autolytic, enzymatic, conservative sharp, sharp, and surgical. It is important that the clinician who is treating the wound bed knows when surgical intervention is needed. Typically, heel PI can be debrided as long as the patient does not have poor perfusion.[26]

Products

- Products that have known safety in infants are amorphous hydrogels, honey dressings, polyhexamethylene biguanide, collagen, 3% bismuth tribromophenate, and petrolatum.[23–25,27,28]

Table 1
Medical device–related pressure injury prevention

Medical Device	Nursing Intervention: For all Ages of Pediatric Patients	Clinician Implementation Tips
Pulse Ox	• Assess skin and rotate digits minimum q8h • If pulse ox is applied to a foot, alternate feet minimum q8h • Patients with poor perfusion, assess skin at the probe site more frequently	• Avoid digit with known PI • Avoid placing on poorly perfused digits
Tracheostomy	• Assess skin with tracheostomy cares • Position the head in a flexed position	• Assess tightness of tracheostomy ties by fitting 1 finger between the ties and neck (notify ENT if too tight due to edema) • Foam dressing with evaporative properties to be applied in the OR under tracheostomy and tracheostomy ties • Apply foam dressing for moisture and redness at the tracheostomy site under the device or ties once matured • Apply wicking fabric/foam under the tracheostomy with moisture present
Continuous positive airway pressure/bilevel positive airway pressure masks and nasal cannulas	• Assess the skin under device q4h or with cares • Alternate mask and prongs q4h if able (nasal, full face, cannula) • Wash mask daily	• Apply No-Sting barrier film MWF and allow to dry with moisture present, before mask application • Patients >1 y use gel or foam dressing to the columella or bridge of the nose with identified erythema
C-Collar	• Assess the skin every shift	• For areas of identified redness, apply foam dressing
Intravenous (IV) hubs/lines	• Assess skin with hourly IV checks • Ensure that the patient is not lying on the IV line or securement device	• Position patient off of lines • If redness is identified under an IV hub, apply a small piece of foam underneath or IV Sponge tape and retape the PIV • If edema noted from tightness of tape, retape

(continued on next page)

Medical Device	Nursing Intervention: For all Ages of Pediatric Patients	Clinician Implementation Tips
Table 1 (*continued*)		
Nasal cannula, NG, NJ, OD, ETT	• Assess the skin under and near the tube q2h with repositioning • Position the lines away from the patient's ears • Assess the lip and mucous membranes under ET tubes with repositioning	• Assess the skin under and near the tube q2h • Position the lines away from the patient's ears
ECMO	• Assess skin around all ECMO cannula sites with skin assessment	• Pad under the lines with a foam dressing with MD agreement
vEEG leads	• Assess skin under leads once removed • Pad the head of immobile patients	• If redness observed, notify provider and electroencephalogram tech; move the lead if possible
ID band	• Assess skin and tightness every shift	• Band should rotate without slipping off
Gastrostomy and GJ tubes	• Assess the skin under and around the stoma every shift	• Use split gauze or foam dressing for padding and moisture wicking under the bumper • If bumper is too tight, notify primary team

Data from Refs.[13,14,21]

- Products to avoid: Calcium phosphate, sustained release silver, and lanolin. Products safe for teenagers and young adults, but avoid in the younger population: methylene blue, gentian viotic, and cadexomer iodine.[23–25,27,28]
- Safe products for older children include: amorphous hydrogel, manuka honey, antimicrobial gauze, alginates, hydrofibers, soft silicone dressings, hydrocolloid, and polymeric membrane.[23–25,27,28] The rate of silver absorption in children is unknown. Products with low levels of silver appear to be safe but should have close clinician oversight.
- Caution should be taken in using antiseptic agents that have been known to cause harm in infants. Products to avoid include alcohols as topical antiseptics, aniline diaper dye, boric acid as a diaper powder, neomycin, povodine-iodine topical antiseptic, sulfa-silvadene, and lidocaine-prolocaine local antiseptic cream.[29]

SUMMARY

PI is a concern in all pediatric critical care populations, and prevention is key. PI prevention efforts must align with the child's physiologic differences in growth and development. An interdisciplinary approach should be instituted for prevention measures.

DISCLOSURE

The author has nothing to disclose.

REFERENCES

1. European Pressure Ulcer Advisory Panel, National Pressure Injury Advisory Panel and Pan Pacific Pressure Injury Alliance. In: Haesler E, editor. Prevention and treatment of pressure ulcers/injuries. EPUAP/NPIAP/PPIA; 2019.
2. Delmore B, Deppisch M, DNurs CS, et al. Pressure injuries in the pediatric population: a national pressure ulcer advisory panel white paper. Adv Skin Wound 2019;32(No. 9):394–408.
3. Kalia YN, Nonato LB, Lund CH, et al. Development of the skin barrier function in premature infants. J Invest Dermatol 1998;111(2):320–6.
4. Lund C, Keller J, lane A, et al. Neonatal skin care: the scientific basis for practice. Neonatal Netw 1999;18(4):15–27.
5. Fuhr JW, Darlenski R, Lachmann N, et al. Infant epidermal skin physiology: adaptation after birth. Br J Dermatol 2011;166:483–90.
6. Manning MJ, Gauvreau K, Curley MA. Factors associated with occipital pressure ulcers in hospitalized infants and children. Am J Crit Care 2015;24(4):342–8.
7. Lyren A, Brille R, Bird M, et al. Ohio Children's Hospitals' solutions for patient safety: a framework for pediatric patient safety improvement. J Healthc Qual 2016;38(No. 4):213–22.
8. Lyren A, Brilli R, Zieker K, et al. Children's Hospitals' solutions for patient safety collaborative impact on hospital-acquired harm. Pediatrics 2017;140(No. 3):e20163494.
9. Fairview patient education: chlorhexidine gluconate (CHG) bathing to prevent new infection; Accessed February 23, 2020.
10. Lund CH, Osborne JW, Kuller J, et al. Neonatal skin care: clinical outcomes of the AWHONN/NANN evidence based clinical practice guideline. Association of the Women's Health, Obstetric and Neonatal Nurses and National Association of Neonatal Nurses. J Obstet Gynecol Neonatal Nurs 2001;30(1):41–51.
11. Wang EW, Layon AJ. Chlorhexidine gluconate use to prevent hospital acquired infections – a use tool, not a panacea. Ann Transl Med 2017;5(1):14.
12. Mayo Clinic. Potty training: how to get the job done. Accessed February 23, 2020.
13. Loo M. Diaper rash (yeast infection). Integrative Medicine for Children 2009.
14. Thompson K, Drummond K, Spencer SM. Nutrition interventions to optimize pediatric wound healing: an evidence-based clinical pathway. Nutr Clin Pract 2014;29(4):473–82.
15. Visscher M, King A, Nie AM, et al. A quality improvement collaborative project to reduce pressure ulcers in PICU's. Pediatrics 2013;131:e1950.
16. Boyer V. Outcomes of a quality improvement program to reduce hospital-acquired pressure ulcers in pediatric patients. Ostomy Wound Manage 2018;64(11):22–8.
17. Altimier, Phillips. Neonatal integrative developmental care model: seven neuroprotective core measures for family-centered developmental care. Neonatal and Infant Reviews 2013;(13):9–22.
18. Kovocs CS. Bone development in the fetus and neonate: role of calciotropic hormones. Curr Osteoporos Rep 2011;9(4):274–83.
19. Visscher M, Lacina L, Casper T, et al. Conformational positioning improves sleep in premature infants with feeding difficulties. J Pediatr 2014;166(1):44–8.

20. Deo Sing C, Shoqirat N. Pressure redistribution crib mattress. J Wound Ostomy Continence Nurs 2019;26(No.1):62–4.
21. American Family Physician. SIDS and safe sleep environment for infants. AAP Update and Recommendations 2017;(12):806–7.
22. McLane KM, Kroskop TA, McCord S, et al. Comparison of interface pressures in the pediatric population among various support surfaces. J Wound ostomy Continence Nurs 2002;29(5):242–51.
23. Bryant R, Nix D. Acute & chronic wounds, current management concepts. 5th edition. Mosby; 2016.
24. Schluer AB, Schols J, halfens R. Pressure ulcer treatment in pediatric patients. Adv Skin Wound Care 2013;25(No. 11):504–10.
25. Black K, Cico SJ, Caglar D. Wound management. Pediatr Rev 2015;35:207.
26. Boesch RP, Myers C, Garrett T, et al. Prevention of tracheostomy related pressure ulcers in children. Pediatrics 2012;129(No 3):e792–7.
27. Boyer V. Treating pediatric pressure injury. Ostomy Wound Manage 2019;65(No. 5):2640–5245.
28. Fox M. Wound care in the neonatal intensive care unit. Neonatal Netw 2011; 30(No. 5):291–303.
29. Mancini A. Skin. Pediatrics 2004;113(3):1114.

Medical Device–Related Pressure Injuries

Joyce Pittman, PhD, RN, ANP-BC, FNP-BC, CWOCN[a],*, Carroll Gillespie, MS, BSN, RN, CWOCN[b]

KEYWORDS

- Medical device–related pressure injury • Pressure injury • Prevention
- Evidence-based practice • Pressure

KEY POINTS

- Common types of medical devices that can cause pressure injuries include respiratory devices, tubes/drains, and compression wraps/splints/braces.
- Pressure injury prevention strategies include: appropriate selection of the correct device, fitting, and securing of the device; pressure redistribution; and prevention bundle strategy.
- Key components of an MDRPI prevention bundle include to: remove device as soon as medically possible, apply prophylactic dressing between device and skin, reposition device frequently, and use a multimodal prevention approach (bundle).

INTRODUCTION

Hospital-acquired pressure injuries (HAPI) occur all too often causing pain, loss of function, infection, extended hospital stay, mortality, and increased costs.[1–3] Despite best practice prevention strategies and advanced technologies, HAPI continue to occur.[4] Recent reports indicate an increase in HAPI[4] with a significant percentage of pressure injuries related to a medical device. Black and colleagues[5] reported that those patients with a medical device were two to four times more likely to develop a pressure injury. Medical device-related pressure injury (MDRPI) prevalence rates in adults range as high as 50%.[5–9]

Before 2016 there was no concise definition of MDRPI for clinicians, which caused confusion when assessing skin injuries and when conducting pressure injury prevalence surveys. In 2015, Pittman and colleagues,[7(pp154)] developed an organizational position statement that defined MDRPI as "a localized injury to the skin and/or underlying tissue including mucous membranes, as a result of pressure, with a history of an external medical device at the location of the ulcer, and mirrors the shape of the device." In 2016, the National Pressure Injury Advisory Panel (NPIAP), formerly the National Pressure Ulcer Advisory Panel, revised their pressure injury staging definitions and provided clarity and an evidence-based definition for MDRPI.[10] NPIAP staging

[a] College of Nursing, University of South Alabama, HAHN 3057, 5721 USA Drive North, Mobile, AL 36688, USA; [b] Arjo, Inc, 2349 West Lake Street, Addison, IL 60101, USA
* Corresponding author.
E-mail address: joycepittman@southalabama.edu

Crit Care Nurs Clin N Am 32 (2020) 533–542
https://doi.org/10.1016/j.cnc.2020.08.004
0899-5885/20/© 2020 Elsevier Inc. All rights reserved.

revision states, "medical device related pressure injuries result from the use of devices designed and applied for diagnostic or therapeutic purposes. The resultant pressure injury generally conforms to the pattern or shape of the device. The injury should be staged using the staging system."[10(pg595)] The NPIAP staging system provides classification of the injury according to the depth of the skin damage. However, in some cases, devices can cause pressure injuries on mucosal membranes and these cannot be classified using the staging classification terminology because of difference in the mucosal membrane anatomic structure. These should be identified as mucosal membrane device-related pressure injury.[1,10]

Until recently, MDRPI were not consistently nor systematically identified or measured when conducting pressure injury surveillance nor included in benchmarking data. However, in 2017, the National Database for Nursing Quality Indicators adopted the NPIAP MDRPI definition and included MDRPI in their pressure injury data collection definitions.[11] National Database for Nursing Quality Indicators inclusion of MDRPI provides clear expectations for benchmarking and supports identification and prevention initiatives targeted toward MDRPI.

In 2019, the International Clinical Practice Guideline[1] for pressure injuries expanded the definition of MDRPIs to include those devices used for diagnostic or therapeutic reasons but also nonmedical devices, such as bed clutter, furniture, and equipment. The Guideline lists a multitude of devices often associated with development of pressure injuries. The most common devices that can cause pressure-related injury include respiratory devices, orthopedic devices, urinary/fecal devices, nasogastric/feeding tubes, and a multitude of other devices intended to treat and manage illness.[1] Arnold-Long and colleagues[6] report three main categories of medical devices most commonly associated with pressure injuries: (1) respiratory devices, (2) tubes/drains, and (3) compression warps/splints/braces. Using these categories of medical devices, this article provides evidence-based information regarding the most common devices that cause pressure injuries in adults and describes current best evidence-based prevention strategies.

RESPIRATORY DEVICES

Chronic and acute medical illnesses often require the use of a respiratory device for intensive management of the condition. The use of respiratory devices, such as endotracheal tubes, is found primarily in the acute care setting but a variety of respiratory devices are also used across care settings. Respiratory devices include, but are not limited to, oxygen delivery and monitoring systems, such as endotracheal tubes, nasal cannulas, continuous positive airway pressure/bilevel positive airway pressure (CPAP/BIPAP) masks, and oxygen tubing; oxygen saturation monitoring devices; and tracheostomy faceplate and securement devices (**Table 1**). Arnold-Long and colleagues[6] reported 10% to 71% incidence of MDRPI related to oxygen tubing and CPAP/BIPAP devices. Kayser and colleagues[8] reported in their retrospective analysis of 102,865 patients, up to 35% of MDRPI were related to respiratory devices (oxygen tubes and CPAP/BIPAP masks). The most common location for MDRPI in these studies was on the ears (29% to 35%).[5,8] The evidence strongly suggests respiratory devices are a risk factor for development of a pressure injury and preventive strategies should be considered.

TUBES/DRAINS

Tubes and drains are another common type of medical device that can cause a pressure injury. Any tube or drain inserted into a body orifice or surgically created opening

Table 1
Device types

Category	Device
Respiratory devices	Nasal cannula/tubing
	BIPAP/CPAP
	Oxygen delivery masks
	Endotracheal tubes/holders/ties
	Tracheostomy tube flange/ties
	Oxygen-sensing monitoring devices (pulse oximeter)
Tubes/drains	Nasogastric tubes/percutaneous endoscopic gastrostomy tubes
	Foley catheters
	Arterial lines, central lines, intravenous catheters/tubing
	Fecal containment devices
	Chest tubes
	Surgical drains
	Rectal probes
Compression wraps/splints/braces	Venous stasis wraps
	Heel protectors
	Deep vein thrombosis sleeves/tubing
	Cervical collars
	Thoracic lumbar sacral orthosis brace
	Cast
	Fracture splints/immobilizers
	Thromboembolic-deterrent stockings
	Blood pressure cuffs
Miscellaneous	Electroencephalogram leads
	Bedpans, urinals

has the potential to cause a pressure injury on the adjacent tissue. The damage could be on skin or mucosal membranes and should be staged accordingly. Tubes and drains include devices, such as, but not limited to, urinary/fecal catheters, nasogastric tubes, gastrostomy tubes, surgical drains, chest tubes, central venous and dialysis catheters, and intravenous catheters (see **Table 1**).

Although there are several studies reporting prevalence of MDRPI, there is variation in study design. Many studies report the MDRPI by body location, and by specific device but do not classify the device into type, creating challenges in summarizing the data. Prevalence of MDRPI caused by nasogastric tubes has been reported by Ambutas and colleagues[12] as 23%, and Arnold-Long and colleagues[6] reported 17% of MDRPI were caused by urinary/fecal tubes. Coyer and colleagues[13] reported 3.1% prevalence (15/483) of MDRPI with 8 of the 15 caused by nasogastric tubes (53%). The evidence indicates tubes and drains are a risk factor for development of a pressure injury and when present, pressure preventive strategies should be considered.

COMPRESSION WRAPS/SPLINTS/BRACES

Management of medical conditions, such as venous stasis disease, lymphedema, and congestive heart failure, often necessitates the use of compression wraps or garments to control lower or upper extremity edema. Prevention of deep vein thrombosis necessitates the use of compression devices. Any compression wrap, garment, or device can lead to development of pressure injuries. External pressure from splints and braces that are applied for fractures or realignment of deformities can also cause pressure injury development. Kayser and colleagues[8] reported prevalence of MDRPI from sequential compression devices was 7.7% and cast/splints was 12%. Arnold-Long and colleagues[6] found 17% of MDRPI were caused by splints, braces, and boots. Powers and colleagues[14] in their study of 484 patients with a cervical collar, noted 6.8% developed a pressure injury. Apold and Rydrych[15] reported the most common type of devices causing MDRPI were cervical collars (22%), immobilizers (17%), and stockings/boots (12%). Black and colleagues,[5] reported MDRPI prevalence by body location but reported device type on a case-by-case basis. These investigators identified one MDRPI on the hand from a brace, one on the occiput from a neck collar, and one on the heel from antiembolism hose. Ham and colleagues[16] examined pressure injuries in trauma patients with suspected spine injury. Of the 145 pressure injuries, 39% were related to devices and 61% were caused by immobilizing devices.[16] Evidence demonstrates that external pressure from splints/braces is one primary cause of MDRPI and should be considered as a risk factor for development of a pressure injury.

MEDICAL DEVICE–RELATED PRESSURE INJURY PREVENTION STRATEGIES

Prevention strategies are imperative to decreasing the number of HAPI and have been implemented in most health care settings. The 5 million Lives Campaign by the Institute for Healthcare Improvement recommends "preventing pressure injuries by reliably using science-based guidelines for their prevention."[17(pp481)] The 2019 Pressure Ulcer/Injury Prevention and Treatment Clinical Practice Guideline[1] provides evidence-based recommendations for pressure injury prevention. Key elements of a pressure injury prevention program include: (1) skin and soft tissue assessment on admission for all patients, (2) an individualized risk assessment for patients, (3) skin and soft tissue assessment routinely, (4) moisture management, (5) nutrition and hydration optimization, and (6) minimization of pressure.[18] Although these strategies are important, they are aimed to prevent nondevice-related pressure injuries and not specifically for device-related pressure injuries. In addition to the previously mentioned strategies, there are three main broad prevention categories for MDRPI shown in the literature: (1) appropriate selection, fitting, and securing of the device[1,15,16,19]; (2) pressure redistribution[1,19–23]; and (3) prevention bundles.[15,16,19,20] Specific prevention strategies are discussed next (**Box 1**).

Appropriate Selection, Fitting, and Securing of the Device

There is a variety of evidence demonstrating effective prevention strategies but most are for specific devices, making it challenging to generalize across devices. The 2019 Clinical Practice Guideline provides an overview of the most current evidence related to MDRPI,[1] and states medical device design, shape, and fitting are associated with MDRPIs.[1]

When selecting the device to be used, the health care professional should consider the appropriate selection, fit, and securement of the device.[1] The most appropriate device (rigid vs flexible) should be selected to meet the needs of the patient and the device should be removed as soon as medically possible.[1] Ackland and colleagues[24] found the risk of an MDRPI caused by a cervical collar increased 66% for every 1 day in the collar. The 2019 Clinical Practice Guideline[1] recommends a trained health care professional should consider several things when choosing a device: the device's ability to minimize tissue damage, correct sizing/shape of the device for the individual, ability to follow manufacturer instructions when applying the device, and the ability

> **Box 1**
> **Medical device–related pressure injury prevention strategies**
>
> Appropriate Selection, Fitting, and Securing of the Device
> - Choose the most appropriate device that meets the patient's need (rigid vs flexible)
> - Remove the device as soon as medically possible
> - Ensure the correct sizing/shape of the device to the individual
> - Correctly apply the device according to the manufacturer's instructions
> - Regularly monitor the tension of medical device securements
> - Instruct patient to notify staff for discomfort at device site
> - Assess the skin under and around the medical device for signs of pressure as part of a routine skin assessment
> - As the patient conditions change, reassess device for correct fit (edema)
> - Secure the device to prevent movement, pressure, and dislodgement; consider the use of commercially available securement devices
> - Follow manufacturers guidelines for indications, monitoring, removal for device
>
> Pressure Redistribution
> - Reposition or regularly rotate the device frequently
> - Apply a prophylactic dressing between the device and skin
> - Avoid positioning a patient directly on top of a medical device
> - Consider the gravitational pull of the device on the surrounding tissues and minimize pressure on those adjacent tissues
> - Remove device when appropriate
> - Alternate the oxygen delivery device (mask vs nasal prongs)
> - Replace rigid extrication cervical collar with a more flexible collar as soon as possible
>
> Prevention Bundles
> - Communicate shift to shift the plan of care regarding medical device and prevention
>
> Tracheostomy Bundle[19]
> - Prophylactic dressing (hydrocolloid) immediate postsurgery
> - Suture removal after 7 days
> - Prophylactic dressing (foam)
> - Neutral positioning of the head
>
> Cervical Collar[15]
> - Obtain and monitor correct cervical collar and fit
> - Decrease prolonged pressure through removal of device or repositioning
> - Routine skin assessment, provide skin and collar care
> - Patient and family education
>
> General MDRPI Bundle[31]
> - Remove device as soon as medically possible
> - Apply prophylactic dressing between device and skin
> - Reposition device frequently
> - Use a multimodal approach (bundle)
>
> *Data from Refs.*[15,19,31]

to correctly secure the device. In addition, the tension of the medical device securements should be monitored. The device should be removed to minimize pressure or adjusted frequently to perform a thorough skin assessment under the device.[1] Apold and Rydrych[15] found most MDRPI (63%) had no documentation of device removal or skin inspection under the device. Ham and colleagues[16] incorporated daily skin care around and under the device and application of cotton stockings underneath the cervical collar for moisture absorption and to optimize skin condition (see **Box 1**).

Consider innovative practices that may minimize pressure on the adjacent skin. One such practice is the "I-tape" method to secure a nasogastric tube. Two direct-care nurses in the critical care unit of a large Midwest health care organization participated in the American Association of Critical Care Nurses Clinical Scene Investigator Academy in 2013 and developed this method.[25] It is a simple use of cloth tape cut strategically to secure the tube to the nose without causing pressure-related skin damage.

The appropriate size and fit of the device must be considered. The device's characteristics (rigidity and material) and/or the patients changing condition (edema) must be considered and monitored. This is especially important for oxygen delivery devices on the face. The 2019 Clinical Practice Guideline[1] recommends alternating the oxygen delivery nasal prongs and a correctly fitted mask device. Implementation tools that incorporate best evidence are helpful to guide prevention and act as a quick reference for clinicians at the bedside. An algorithm to guide prevention of MDRPI caused by respiratory devices was developed by an interdisciplinary group of direct-care nurses, respiratory technicians, clinical nurse specialist, and wound, ostomy, continence nurses at a large Midwest health care organization. The purpose of this tool was to guide clinicians in prevention of respiratory MDRPI (**Fig. 1**).[26]

Pressure Redistribution

Pressure redistribution is a fundamental strategy for pressure injury prevention. This strategy is also true for MDRPI. Redistribution of pressure caused by a medical device is accomplished by repositioning the device frequently or by providing a prophylactic dressing between the device and skin. The 2019 Clinical Practice Guideline provides a Good Practice Statement, which states to regularly rotate or reposition the medical device and provide support for the device to minimize pressure.[1] Clinically, this means the nurse should consider the location of the device, reposition it frequently, and/or position the patient so they are not laying directly on the device if possible. Also, consider the gravitational pull of the device on the surrounding tissues and minimize pressure on those adjacent tissues. This is done by supporting the device away from the skin or alternating the direction of the mechanical force of the device frequently. For example, if the ventilation equipment is on the right side of the patient and the tubing is exerting pressure on the right side of the tracheal collar, consider moving the ventilation machine to the left side of the patient to minimize pressure of the tube on the skin. Another example is the use of stabilizing devices to support the medical device, such as the bumper on the gastrostomy tube that keeps the tube upright and not laying directly on the skin.

There is direct evidence demonstrating the effectiveness of prophylactic dressings to reduce MDRPI. A variety of types of prophylactic dressings have been examined: hydrocolloid, foam, silicone gel, and transparent dressings. Each type of prophylactic dressing may differ in their properties and qualities and it is important to consider the needs of the patient when selecting the type of prophylactic dressing. For example, some dressings are designed to adhere well to the skin, whereas others have more absorptive properties. Using a prophylactic dressing has been shown to be effective in reducing MDRPI for tracheostomies,[19] endotracheal tubes,[27] ventilation prongs and masks,[28,29] and under casts.[23] However, in a systematic review by Clark and colleagues,[21] no specific type of prophylactic dressing was found to be more effective than another (see **Box 1**).[21]

Prevention Bundles

Evidence-based prevention in the health care setting often involves using a care bundle approach. A bundle approach refers to a set of interventions designed to prevent the occurrence of a condition or complication. Using a bundle approach has been shown to be effective in preventing ventilator-associated pneumonia, catheter-associated urinary tract infections, and a multitude of other conditions.[30] A variety

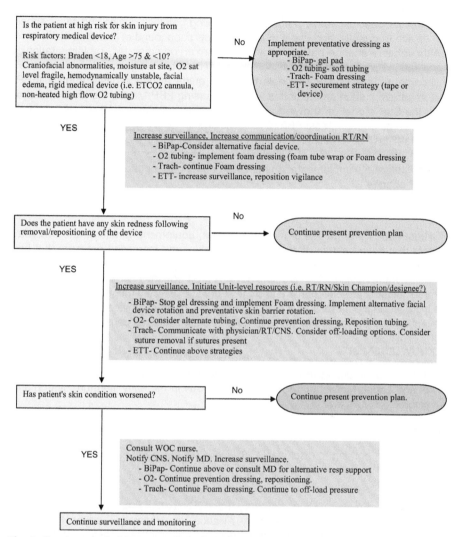

Fig. 1. Respiratory decision tree. CNS, clinical nurse specialist; ETT, endotracheal tube; RT, respiratory technician; WOC, wound, ostomy, continence. (*Courtesy of* Joyce Pittman, PhD, RN, ANP-BC, FNP-BC, CWOCN, FAAN, Mobile, AL.)

of prevention bundles have been shown to be effective in reducing MDRPI. O'Toole and colleagues[19] describe a prevention bundle for tracheostomies that includes: prophylactic dressing (hydrocolloid) immediate postsurgery, suture removal after 7 days, prophylactic dressing (foam), and neutral positioning of the head. Black and colleagues[20] provide general recommendations for MDRPI: prophylactic dressing (foam) between the device and skin, repositioning of the device frequently, and do not add more padding if device is tight. Apold and Rydrych[15] recommend a prevention bundle for cervical collars that includes: obtain and monitor correct cervical collar and fit, decrease prolonged pressure through removal of device or repositioning and assessment, skin and collar care, and patient and family education. To summarize, prevention bundle recommendations for MDRPI include to: remove device as soon as medically possible, apply prophylactic dressing between device and skin, reposition device frequently, and use a multimodal approach (bundle) (see **Box 1**).[31]

Although an evidence-based bundle approach is recommended, implementation of a prevention bundle may be insufficient in and of itself to change practice in a complex environment. There several models that help guide evidence-base practice (EBP) implementation, such as the Johns Hopkins Nursing EBP Model, the Iowa Model of EBP, the Star Model of Knowledge Transformation, the Ottawa Model of Research Use, and many others. Most EBP models include the following components or a variation that must be considered when implementing EBP: the innovation evidence, practice environment, key stakeholders (clinicians and patients) or team, barriers and facilitators, an implementation plan, and continued monitoring and evaluation of the EBP change.

SUMMARY

MDRPIs result from the use of medical devices, equipment, furniture, and everyday objects that have been in direct contact with skin, and increased pressure that has caused soft tissue damage.[1] The resultant pressure injury generally mirrors the pattern or shape of the device.[7-10,31] Medical devices are frequently necessary in the current complex health care environment and the nurse and clinician must be hypervigilant of the increased risk of pressure injuries with the use of these devices. Evidence-based prevention strategies are key to minimizing the harm devices can cause.

ACKNOWLEDGMENTS

The authors gratefully acknowledge the contributions of Janet Cuddigan, PhD, RN, FAAN and Laurie McNichol, MSN, CWOCN, FAAN in the early literature search and development of this article.

DISCLOSURE

J. Pittman has nothing to disclose. C. Gillespie is employed at Arjo, Inc.

REFERENCES

1. European Pressure Ulcer Advisory Panel, National Pressure Injury Advisory Panel, Pan Pacific Pressure Injury Alliance. In: Haesler E, editor. Prevention and treatment of pressure ulcers/injuries: clinical practice guideline. The International guideline. EPUAP/NPIAP/PPPIA; 2019.
2. Pittman J, Beeson T, Dillon J, et al. Hospital Acquired Pressure Injuries and Acute Skin Failure in Critical Car: A Case-Control Study. Journal of Wound Ostomy and Continence Nursing 2020. Pending publication.
3. Song Y, Shen H, Cai J, et al. The relationship between pressure injury complication and mortality risk of older patients in follow-up: a systematic review and meta-analysis. Int Wound J 2019;16(6):1533–44.
4. AHRQ. Types of health care quality measures. Agency for Healthcare Research and Quality. Available at: https://www.ahrq.gov/talkingquality/measures/types.html. Accessed October 7, 2019.
5. Black J, Cuddigan J, Walko M, et al. Medical device related pressure ulcers in hospitalized patients. Int Wound J 2010;7(5):358–65.
6. Arnold-Long M, Ayer M, Borchert K. Medical device-related pressure injuries in long-term acute care hospital setting. J Wound Ostomy Continence Nurs 2017; 44(4):325–30.

7. Pittman J, Beeson T, Kitterman J, et al. Medical device-related hospital-acquired pressure ulcers: development of an evidence-based position statement. J Wound Ostomy Continence Nurs 2015;42(2):151–4.

8. Kayser S, VanGilder C, Ayello E, et al. Prevalence and analysis of medical device-related pressure injuries: results from the international pressure ulcer prevalence surveey. Adv Skin Wound Care 2018;31(6):276–86.

9. Pittman J, Beeson T, Dillon J, et al. Hospital-acquired pressure injuries in critical and progressive care: avoidable versus unavoidable. Am J Crit Care 2019;28(5): 338–50.

10. Edsberg L, Black J, Goldberg M, et al. Revised National Pressure Ulcer Advisory Panel pressure injury staging system. J Wound Ostomy Continence Nurs 2016; 43(6):585–97.

11. NDNQI. Guidelines for data collection and submission on pressure injury indicator. Overland Park (KS): Press Ganey; 2017.

12. Ambutas S, Staffileno B, Fogg L. Reducing nasal pressure ulcers with an alternative taping device. Medsurg Nurs 2014;23(2):96–100.

13. Coyer F, Stotts N, Blackman V. A prospective window into medical device-related pressure ulcers in intensive care. Int Wound J 2014;11(6):656–64.

14. Powers J, Daniels D, McGuire C, et al. The incidence of skin breakdown associated with use of cervical collars. J Trauma Nurs 2006;13(4):198–200.

15. Apold J, Rydrych D. Preventing device-related pressure ulcers: using data to guide statewide change. J Nurs Care Qual 2012;27(1):28–34.

16. Ham W, Schoonhoven L, Schuurmans M, et al. Pressure ulcers in trauma patients with suspected spine injury: a prospective cohort study with emphasis on device-related pressure ulcers. Int Wound J 2016;160:D371.

17. McCannon CJ, Hackbarth A, Griffin F. Miles to go: an introduction to the 5 million Lives Campaign. Joint Comm J Qual Patient Saf 2007;33(8):477–84.

18. Duncan K. Preventing pressure ulcers: the goal is zero. Joint Comm J Qual Patient Saf 2007;33(10):605–10.

19. O'Toole T, Jacobs N, Hondorp B, et al. Prevention of tracheostomy-related hospital-acquired pressure ulcers. Otolaryngol Head Neck Surg 2017;156(4):642–51.

20. Black J, Alves P, Brindle CT, et al. Use of wound dressings to enhance prevention of pressure ulcers caused by medical devices. Int Wound J 2015;12(3):322–7.

21. Clark M, Black J, Alves P, et al. Systematic review of the use of prophylactic dressings in the prevention of pressure ulcers. Int Wound J 2014;11:460–71.

22. Zibari GB, Boykin KN, Sawaya DE, et al. Pancreatic transplantation and subsequent graft surveillance by pancreatic portal-enteric anastomosis and temporary venting jejunostomy. Ann Surg 2001;233(5):639–44.

23. Forni C, Loro L, Tremosini M, et al. Use of polyurethane foam inside plaster casts to prevent onset of heel sores in the population at risk. A controlled study. J Clin Nurs 2011;20(5/6):675–80.

24. Ackland HM, Cooper DJ, Malham GM, et al. Factors predicting cervical collar-related decubitus ulceration in major trauma patients. Spine 2007;32(4):423–8.

25. Markowitz J, Spurgeon H. Face the pressure: reducing device-related pressure ulcers. AACN; 2013.

26. Pittman J, Beeson T. Device-related pressure injury task force. Respiratory decision tree. Indiana University Health Academic Health Center; 2017.

27. Whitley A, Nygaard R, Endorf F. Reduction of pressure-related complications with an improved method of securing endotracheal tubes in burn patients with facial burns. J Burn Care Res 2018;31.

28. Weng M. The effect of protective treatment in reducing pressure ulcers for non-invasive ventilation patients. Intensive Crit Care Nurs 2008;24(5):295–9.
29. Huang T, Tseng C, Lee T, et al. Preventing pressure sores of the nasal ala after nasotracheal tube intubation: from animal model to clinical application. J Oral Maxillofac Surg 2009;67:543–51.
30. Tayyib N, Coyer F. Translating pressure ulcer prevention into intensive care: nursing practice overlaying a care bundle approach with a model for Research implementation. J Nurs Care Qual 2017;32(1):6–14.
31. Pittman J. NPUAP Medical Device-Related Pressure Injury. Oral presentation NPUAP Annual Conference. National Pressure Ulcer Advisory Panel. Las Vegas, NV: Aria Hotel; 2018.

Unstageable Pressure Injuries

Identification, Treatment, and Outcomes Among Critical Care Patients

Sunniva Zaratkiewicz, PhD, RN, CWCN*,
Mark Goetcheus, BSN, RN, CWON, CFCN, CDE,
Holly Vance, BSN, RN, CWON

KEYWORDS

- Unstageable • Pressure injuries • Pressure ulcers • Slough • Eschar

KEY POINTS

- Unstageable pressure injuries can be challenging for health care professionals to correctly identify, despite refinement of staging definitions and interventions designed to improve correct identification.
- Treatment of unstageable pressure injuries in the critical care setting varies, with some of these wounds healing by secondary intention after selective débridement and others requiring surgical interventions and musculocutaneous flaps for closure.
- A key component in the treatment of unstageable pressure injuries is débridement. Understanding the multiple types of selective and nonselective débridement is essential to the creation of a patient-centered, individualized wound care plan.
- Although the body of literature on unstageable pressure injuries has grown, there remains much that is not known and further research on these pressure injuries is indicated.

INTRODUCTION

The current widely accepted definition of unstageable pressure injuries (PIs) is that of a full-thickness PI in which the depth is unknown due to a wound base that is covered by slough, which may be yellow, tan, gray, green, or brown, and/or eschar, which may be tan, brown, or black.[1] Until the eschar and/or slough is removed, the true depth and stage cannot be determined.[1,2] Once the slough and/or eschar is débrided, the PI then is staged according to the structures revealed.

While unstageable PIs have likely existed since the dawn of humankind, early documentation can be found in medical texts from the late 1800s in the work of Jean-Martin Charcot x 2.[3] While the National Pressure Injury Advisory Panel (NPIAP), then known

Harborview Medical Center, Box 359733, Seattle, WA 98104, USA
* Corresponding author.
E-mail address: sunnivaz@uw.edu

Crit Care Nurs Clin N Am 32 (2020) 543–561
https://doi.org/10.1016/j.cnc.2020.08.005
0899-5885/20/© 2020 Elsevier Inc. All rights reserved.

as the National Pressure Ulcer Advisory Panel, had a category of unstageable in 1989, the definition at that time referred to "full thickness skin loss – no limit to the damage."[4] The NPAIP refined the definition of unstageable PIs to include the presence of eschar and slough in 2007 with the release of an updated staging system.[5] Since that time unstageable PIs have garnered more attention clinically and from a regulatory perspective. Clinically, these PIs can be challenging to appropriately identify and, at this time, the development of unstageable PIs in hospital settings leads to punitive policies, including public reporting and reduced payments from insurers.[6] This article discusses the current state of the science of unstageable PIs in the critical care setting; their identification, treatment, and outcomes.

CLINICAL PRESENTATION

The earliest evidence of PIs can be found in Egyptian mummies dating back thousands of years.[7] Although unstageable PIs likely existed at that time, one of the earliest published descriptions of these wounds dates back to 1877 when neurologist, Jean-Martin Charcot x 2, described eschar on bed sores (an early synonym for PIs).[3] Charcot included illustrations with his writings (**Figs. 1** and **2**) that visually are consistent with what currently is defined as unstageable PIs, presenting with eschar covering the wound base.

Approximately 150 years later, the clinical presentation of these wounds is much the same, but understanding of the etiology of PIs has advanced significantly and the classification system for PIs has been improved on.

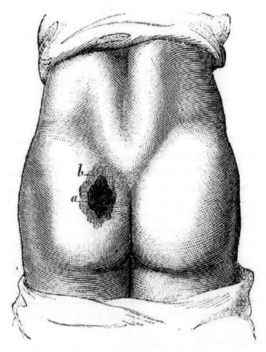

Fig. 1. Lesion over L buttock. (*From* Charcot, JM. Disorders of nutrition consecutive on lesions of the spinal cord and brain. In: Lectures on the diseases of the nervous system, delivered at La Salpetriere. Vol. 1. London, UK: The New Syndenham Society; 1877.)

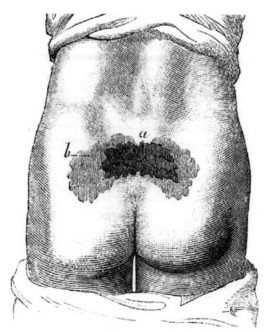

Fig. 2. Lesion over sacrum. (*From* Charcot, JM. Disorders of nutrition consecutive on lesions of the spinal cord and brain. In: Lectures on the diseases of the nervous system, delivered at La Salpetriere. Vol. 1. London, UK: The New Syndenham Society; 1877.)

The NPIAP, the European Pressure Ulcer Advisory Panel, and the Pan Pacific Pressure Injury Alliance jointly define unstageable PIs as "Full-thickness skin and tissue loss in which the extent of tissue damage within the ulcer cannot be confirmed because it is obscured by slough or eschar. If slough or eschar is removed, a stage 3 or stage 4 PI will be revealed. Stable eschar (ie, dry, adherent, intact without erythema or fluctuance) on the heel or ischemic limb should not be softened or removed"[1] (**Figs. 3** and **4**).

Clinical Challenges

Several challenges exist in relation to the definition and staging of unstageable PIs. The following sections recognize specific gaps in the science that would benefit from further research and subsequently improve understanding of unstageable PIs, related patient care, and outcomes.

Definition

Although there have been advancements in PI staging, opportunity exists to enhance current definitions. A 2015 study found 33.8% of unstageable PIs (n = 74) in a level 1 trauma, burn, and safety net hospital and academic medical center healed consistently with partial-thickness wounds.[6] A subsequent study in this setting found 54.2% of unstageable PIs healed consistently with partial-thickness wounds (n = 120).[8] These outcomes suggest a need for further study and a reconsideration of the current definition, which refers to all unstageable PIs as full-thickness wounds.

Staging

Despite the advancements in the state of the science of unstageable PIs, challenges in correct staging by clinicians persist. In a study designed to evaluate the effectiveness

Unstageable Pressure Injury - Dark Eschar

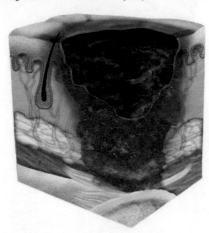

Fig. 3. Unstageable Pressure Injury – Dark Eschar. NPIAP illustrations of PIs. (Used with permission of the National Pressure Injury Advisory Panel on January 21, 2020.)

of PI classification education, a convenience sample, including 407 nurses, found education did not improve visual diagnostic ability to correctly stage unstageable PIs.[9] Another study, which introduced a computerized clinical decision support program with the goal of improving nurses' accuracy when staging PIs, found unstageable and stage 3 PIs were the least frequently correctly staged of all categories, with an overall accuracy of 39%.[10] Studies involving physicians show similar outcomes with participants in a study correctly identifying unstageable PIs only 20% of the time and another reporting physicians' mean scores in PI identification lower than nurses' (69% vs 76%, respectively), with just 45% of physicians in this study able to correctly identify unstageable PIs.[11,12]

Unstageable Pressure Injury - Slough and Eschar

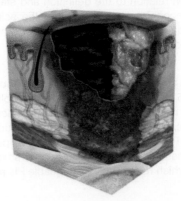

Fig. 4. Unstageable Pressure Injury – Sough and Eschar. NPIAP illustrations of PIs. (Used with permission of the National Pressure Injury Advisory Panel on January 21, 2020.)

Slough and eschar

The hallmark property of unstageable PIs is the presence of slough and/or eschar. Given that PIs are staged according to what tissues and structures are visualized in the wound bed, it is necessary that the clinician can identify them correctly for accurate staging to occur. Unfortunately, in clinical practice, slough can be mistaken for surgical mesh, residue from medicinal honey, staining from topical iodine, bone, tendon, or callous.[6,8] Eschar also poses identification challenges and can be mistaken for scabs, crusts, dried blood, and sutures.[6,8] Additionally, the authors of this article have observed black tar heroin residue in wound beds mistaken for eschar.

Assessment

The parameters for clinical assessment of unstageable PIs are consistent with the parameters for assessment of all wounds and include the following elements: etiology (if known), anatomic location, size (length, width, depth, tunneling, and undermining), classification (include staging, in cases of PIs), wound base, wound edges, exudate (include type and amount), signs/symptoms of infection, odor, periwound skin, and associated pain.[13] Additional considerations include ensuring the patient is in the same position for each wound assessment. Consistent positioning of the patient with each wound assessment helps prevent discrepancies in wound size that can occur secondary to the shifting of soft tissues with changes in patient positioning.

TREATMENT OF UNSTAGEABLE PRESSURE INJURIES

Treatment guidelines specific to unstageable PIs vary in the literature; however, the principles of wound bed preparation are always applicable; these include tissue management, infection and inflammation control, moisture balance, epithelial edge advancement, repair and regeneration, and social or other factors related to the patient.[14] Wound care treatment plans for unstageable PIs are multifaceted and work best within an interdisciplinary team approach. If able to participate, the engagement of the patient and family is an integral part in the establishment of appropriate goals of care. Wound and skin treatment, pressure redistribution through repositioning, and appropriate surface selection, pain management, nutrition, and education are key components of any PI treatment plan.[1] PI treatment goals in the critical care setting should be patient-specific and can vary from comfort care measures to surgical interventions. Comprehensive wound care plans are guided by multiple considerations, including, but not limited to, risk and benefit of the treatment, the patient's goals and clinical condition, and expected outcomes.

Débridement

The nonviable tissue of an unstageable PI hinders wound healing, and a débridement plan is necessary for the attainment of a clean wound bed. Facilitating the removal of devitalized tissue enhances the healing process. PIs on anatomic locations with poor perfusion and those on the heels or on ischemic limbs with dry, stable eschar and without signs of infection should not be débrided.[15] In the authors' experiences, this also applies to craniotomy patients who develop unstageable PIs on the head in areas where bone has been removed, because débridement of these areas risks exposure of the brain and other fragile structures. In such scenarios, clinicians should work closely with their neurosurgery colleagues and occupational therapists involved in helmet creation and revisions to ensure the best possible outcomes for the patient.

The information presented in this article includes examples of débridement methods. Consult your state practice acts and facility specific policies to ensure you are working within your scope of practice.

Types of débridement

- Selective débridement involves removal of devitalized tissue exclusively, keeping healthy tissue intact.
- Nonselective débridement involves removal of both viable and nonviable tissues to achieve a clean wound bed.

Types of selective débridement

Autolysis Autolysis is a débridement process utilizing the patient's own white blood cells and enzymes during the inflammation process to break up devitalized tissue naturally.[13] The use of dressings that maintain or create a moist wound environment can assist with autolytic removal of devitalized tissue while preserving viable tissue. Depending on the amount of wound exudate and dressing change frequency, there are a variety of dressing types that can facilitate autolysis, including foam, moist gauze, hydrofibers, alginates, and hydrocolloids. Honey can facilitate autolytic débridement due to the dressing's osmotic pull of the periwound's lymph fluid.[13]

Enzymes Proteolytic enzymes can help with selective removal of devitalized tissue as a débriding agent. Currently, there is only 1 enzymatic débriding agent available, which is derived from *Clostridium* bacteria. The topical enzyme assists with breaking down the collagen's peptide bonds to the necrotic tissue.[16]

Biosurgical/Maggot This biological method of selective débridement utilizes sterile maggots applied within the wound bed. Digestion of devitalized tissue is facilitated by enzymes produced by the maggots.[15]

Chemical Sodium hypochlorite, also known as Dakin solution, commonly is utilized as an antimicrobial agent but also is used clinically to facilitate débridement because the chemical agents may help break down necrotic tissue bonds.

Ultrasound The ultrasound débridement method utilizes acoustic energy to lift devitalized tissue. Some ultrasound débridement treatments are accompanied with saline.[15]

Conservative sharp débridement Conservative sharp debridement involved utilization of sharp instruments, such as scalpels, curettes, and scissors, to remove devitalized tissue only. This débridement technique should not involve viable tissue[13] (**Fig. 5**).

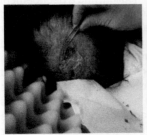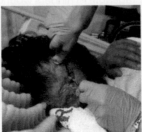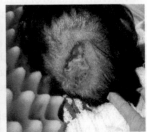

Fig. 5. Conservative sharp débridement of an unstageable PI on occiput.

Types of nonselective débridement

Surgical débridement Surgical débridement involves surgical removal of necrotic tissue to excise the wound bed down to viable tissue, thus transitioning the wound into an acute inflammatory healing phase. It typically is performed in the presence of infection or a significant amount of devitalized tissue.[1]

Wet to dry For wet to dry dressings, moist gauze is applied to a wound, which, once dried and adhered to the wound bed, then is pulled off, with the goal of mechanically removing tissue from the wound bed.

Wound Microbial Bioburden and Infection

Unstageable PIs have a high risk for infection due to the presence of the ischemic tissue.[1] Cleansing at every dressing change is recommended to assist in decreasing bioburden. For wounds with signs of infection and significant necrotic tissue, surgical consultation to evaluate the need for surgical débridement is recommended to expedite the healing process. If the PI is at risk for fecal contamination due to anatomic location, a bowel management program or a fecal management system should be considered. In extreme cases, surgical creation of a diverting colostomy may be appropriate. For PIs with exposed or directly palpable bone, assessment and treatment of osteomyelitis should be considered. In cases of systemic infection, evaluation by a licensed independent provider for appropriate antibiotic therapy is recommended. Antimicrobial dressings as topical agents can assist with the treatment of localized wound infections and reduction of colonization load, thus promoting wound healing. Silver, honey, iodine, sodium hypochlorite, and acetic acid are some examples of common antimicrobial agents embedded in a variety of wound dressings, including gauzes, foams, hydrocolloids, and creams. These antiseptic dressing should be discontinued once the PI transitions to a proliferative stage of healing and is free of signs of infection.

Overly moist warm environments that exist for prolonged periods under dressings are a common cause of cutaneous candidiasis and present as macular and/or papular erythematic rashes with satellite lesions. There is a higher risk of cutaneous candidiasis in patients who are immunocompromised, have a history of corticosteroid therapy, chemotherapy, or recent antibiotic use.[17]

For topical treatment of cutaneous candidiasis, the following should be considered:

- Use of a dressing with properties that help keep the periwound skin dry
- Increasing dressing change frequency or utilizing highly absorptive dressings, such as foams, alginates, or hydrofibers, to assist with maintaining optimum moist wound bed environment while protecting the periwound skin
- Liquid skin sealants, which act as a barrier agent and protect periwound skin from moisture-associated skin damage
- Topical antifungal agents to treat cutaneous fungal infections
- Utilizing the ostomy technique, crusting, in which a liquid skin barrier is used in combination with an antifungal powder, applied in thin layers, and allowed to dry

Dressings

Dressing goals include filling the wound cavity and controlling exudate while maintaining a moist wound environment.[1] To promote the growth of healthy tissue and reduce risk of abscess formation and loculations, the dressing should fill the entirety of the wound bed, including areas of tunneling and undermining. Whenever possible, the use of 1 continuous piece of dressing is encouraged to prevent the occurrence of retained foreign bodies. If the size of the wound and/or presence of tunneling and/

or undermining requires use of multiple pieces of dressings to fill the wound bed, indicate the number of pieces used on the outer dressing and in the wound documentation. This helps to ensure removal of all dressings at the time of each dressing change. Choosing a dressing that controls exudate while keeping the wound bed moist can be challenging and dressing plans may need to be adjusted as the wound evolves. Maintaining healthy periwound skin can assist with wound closure, and use of a skin protectant is helpful in the presence of excessive exudate or repeated use of medical adhesives. Please note that an exhaustive list of dressing brands/types are not included in this article due to an ever-changing and evolving market. These recommendations are meant as general guidelines. For specific dressing indications, refer to manufacturer guidelines.

Gauzes
Gauzes are available in fine mesh and large mesh in multiple sizes. Gauze also is available in rolls and packing strips, which can assist with filling large cavities, tunneling, and undermining. In cases of infection, the use of gauze impregnated with a variety of antimicrobial agents may be considered. Gauzes should be changed daily or more often, because these dressings absorb minimal to moderate exudate.

Hydrocolloids
Hydrocolloids are indicated for minimal to moderate exudate. Hydrocolloids commonly are used as a secondary dressing in combination with wound fillers when there is depth to the wound bed or as primary dressings in the case of shallow wounds. These dressing are designed for multiple-day use.

Foam dressings
Foam dressings available in a variety of shapes and sizes, with and without adhesive borders. Depending on the manufacturer and product, they may be used for moderate to large amounts of drainage and also may be used with wound fillers when there is depth to the wound bed. Foam dressings are indicated for multiple-day use.

Calcium alginate and hydrofibers
Calcium alginate and hydrofiber dressings are indicated for wounds with a large amount of exudate. They are highly absorptive and can act as a wound bed filler. They often require coverage by a secondary dressing, typically a foam or hydrocolloid dressing, and are designed for multiple-day use.

Honey
There are numerous honey products on the market today, including gels, pastes, alginates, and hydrocolloids. Honey helps maintain a moist wound environment and facilitates autolytic and osmotic débridement. Many gels and pastes are indicated to be applied daily, whereas hydrocolloid and alginate dressings are indicated for multiple-day use. The first 2 or 3 applications of honey can increase exudate within the wound beds and, therefore, require more frequent dressing changes initially.

Hydrogels
Hydrogels donate moisture to wound beds and assist in maintaining a moist wound environment. They are indicated for full-thickness and partial-thickness wounds that have minimal to no exudate and may be used with other dressings. Hydrogels come in a variety of forms, including solid dressings and amorphous gels. Dressing change frequency is dependent on the type of hydrogel, ranging from multiple dressing changes per day to multiday indications.[15]

Skin barrier products

Liquid barriers, when applied topically, dry to form a breathable, transparent coating, meant as a prophylactic agent or to treat damaged skin. Skin barriers should be allowed to dry before applying creams, adhesives, or dressings.

Negative-pressure wound therapy

Although commonly used to expedite the healing process, negative-pressure wound therapy (NPWT) historically has not been recommended for use in unstageable PIs due to presence of devitalized tissue in the wound bed. Some new NPWT modalities, however, are indicated for removal of necrotic tissue. Product-specific guidelines should be referred to, to ensure appropriate use.

Pain

Because unstageable PIs can be painful, pain management is an important element in the wound care plan. The plan should address the assessment and management of both prolonged wound pain and pain associated with procedural times, such as dressing changes and débridement.[1] For patients in the critical care setting with cognitive or verbal impairment, pain assessment tools should include nonverbal signs of suspected discomfort, such as facial grimacing, body movements, and changes vital signs.

Offloading the PI with the use of devices and/or repositioning the patient can assist with decreasing wound pain. Additionally, there are numerous nonpharmaceutical approaches to treat pain associated with PIs, including, but not limited to, transcutaneous electric nerve stimulation, virtual reality, and music therapy. A wound care

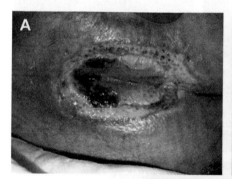
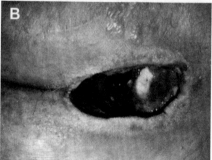
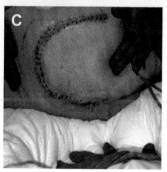

Fig. 6. Unstageable PI in ICU patient, sacrum. (*A*) Prior to debridement. (*B*) Post–surgical débridement. (*C*) After gluteal rotational flap.

plan that decreases the frequency of dressing changes can also reduce episodic pain associated with these procedural events.

Pharmacologic treatment, with the use of systemic analgesics, is common in cases of prolonged wound pain, whereas pain associated with procedures may be treated with systemic and/or topical agents. Topical analgesics, such as lidocaine, come in different forms, including liquids, gels, creams, and patches. Topical analgesic agents that are applied within the wound bed of unstageable PIs may be less effective due to necrotic tissue hindering absorption. In the presence of significant slough and/or eschar in the wound bed, topical anesthetic patches may be applied to the periwound skin. With all pharmaceutical treatments of procedural pain, timing the administration and where the therapeutic onset and peak coincide with the dressing change or débridement procedure should be considered to optimize the therapeutic effect.

Nutrition

Malnutrition and inadequate protein intake have a negative impact on the wound healing process. A nutritional assessment and prompt dietary intervention for patients with unstageable PIs can assist in improving wound healing. Ideally, a nutritionist is a part of the hospital's PI prevention and treatment program.

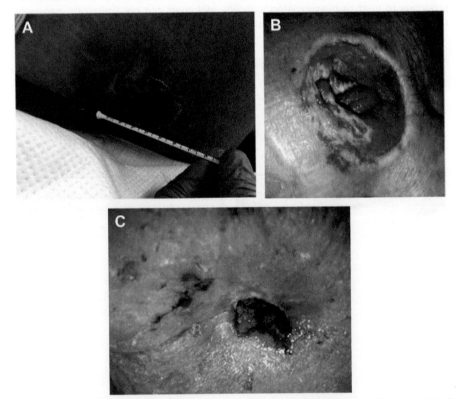

Fig. 7. Unstageable PI in ICU patient, ischium. (*A*) Prior to debridement. (*B*) Post–surgical débridement. (*C*) Wound did not heal.

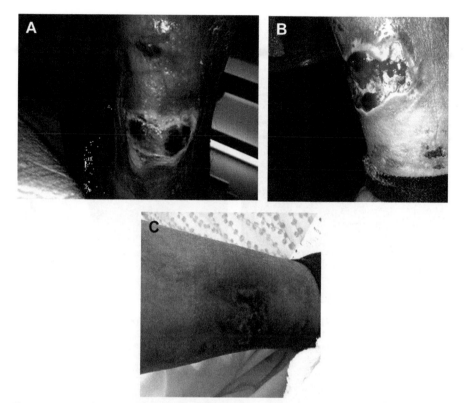

Fig. 8. Unstageable PI in ICU patient, posterior calf. (*A*) Prior to debridement. (*B*) Post–conservative sharp débridement. (*C*) Wound healed by secondary intention.

Support Surfaces and Offloading Devices

Support surfaces, which include mattresses, integrated bed systems, mattress replacements, overlays, seat cushions, and seat cushion overlays, can assist with the treatment of PIs and are a critical part of a wound care plan.[1] Key components of

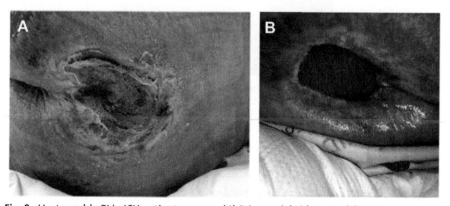

Fig. 9. Unstageable PI in ICU patient, sacrum. (*A*) Prior to debridement. (*B*) Post-conservative sharp debridement.

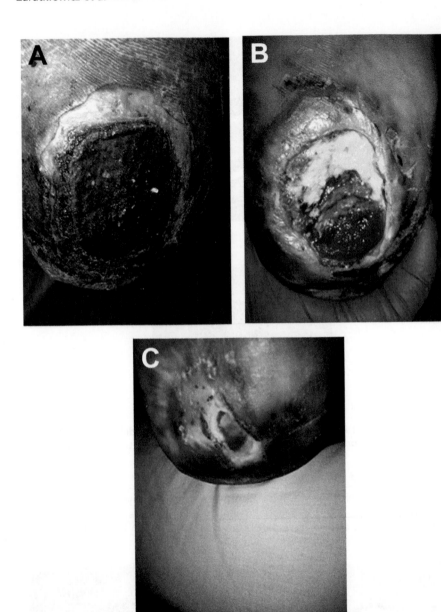

Fig. 10. Unstageable PI in ICU patient, heel. (*A*) Prior to debridement. (*B*) Post–conservative sharp débridement. (*C*) Wound healed by secondary intention.

support surfaces include pressure redistribution and microclimate control.[15] For specific support surface recommendations, utilize the Wound, Ostomy, and Continence Nurses Society support surface algorithm: http://algorithm.wocn.org/#home. This electronic algorithm is available free of charge.

Although specialty surfaces can provide pressure redistribution, they do not replace the need for turning and repositioning.[1] Pressure on the wound bed decreases

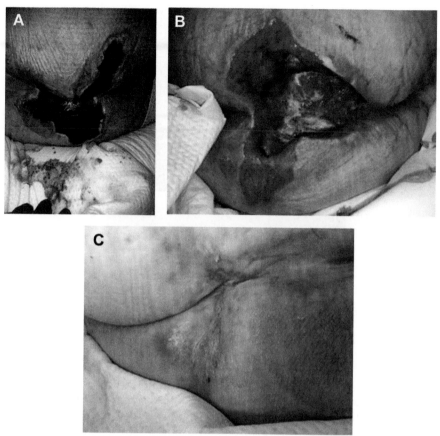

Fig. 11. Unstageable PI in ICU patient, sacrum. (*A*) Prior to debridement. (*B*) Post–surgical débridement. (*C*) Wound healed by secondary intention.

perfusion required for healing; therefore, laying patients directly on wounds should be avoided.

Offloading devices are essential to promote healing of heel PIs. Offloading heel suspension boots or pillows placed under the lower legs are common offloading methods. Ideally, the goal of the offloading device is to keep the heel completed floated, with foot drop prevention properties, and avoiding stress to the Achilles or popliteal vein regions.[1]

For patients who have transitioned to sitting in chairs with unstageable PIs on the buttock region, the wound should be assessed frequently for deterioration, and seating times may need to be restricted to assist with the healing process. A repositioning and offloading schedule should be included in the wound care plan for patients in chairs. Whenever possible, education should be provided to patients, family members, and caregivers on chair sitting offloading techniques. Although pressure redistribution cushions always recommended for patients in chairs, this is especially important for patients who are unable to perform offloading techniques.[1]

OUTCOMES

Among hospitalized patients, those in intensive care units (ICUs) are twice as likely to develop a PI.[18] PIs are associated with unfavorable physical, social, psychosocial, and

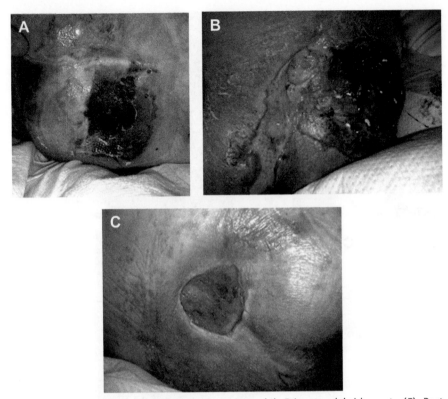

Fig. 12. Unstageable PI in ICU patient, sacrum. (*A*) Prior to debridement. (*B*) Post–conservative sharp débridement. (*C*) Wound did not heal.

economic effects and may lead to negative body image and self-esteem.[19] All of these effects have the power to have an impact on and decrease a patient's quality of life. Due to associated infection and/or need for surgical intervention, the presence of unstageable PIs may increase both length of hospital stay and related health care costs.

Although some patients with unstageable PIs achieve healing by secondary intention after débridement, others may require a musculocutaneous flap to achieve

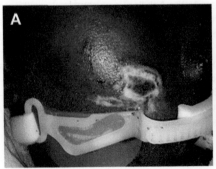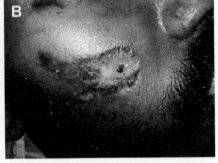

Fig. 13. Unstageable PI in ICU patient, cheek. (*A*) Prior to debridement. (*B*) Wound healed by secondary intention.

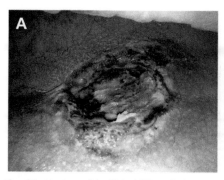 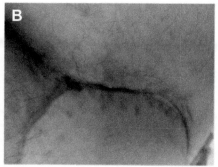

Fig. 14. Unstageable PI in ICU patient, sacrum. (*A*) Post–conservative sharp débridement. Post–surgical débridement. (*B*) Wound healed after gluteal rotational flap intervention.

closure, and some may live with these wounds chronically. Patients with PIs on multiple anatomic turning sites, such as the ischial tuberosities, trochanters, sacrum or coccyx, and other locations, may have limited ability to completely offload their wounds, which further compromises wound healing.

Goals and treatment outcomes for each patient are different and depend on multiple factors. If, after a comprehensive assessment and implementation of recommended interventions, a wound is found to be unlikely to heal, then the goal may be maintenance. Maintenance includes infection prevention, odor and exudate control, minimizing deterioration of the wound bed, and decreasing frequency of dressing changes.[15]

Unavoidable Pressure Injuries

Not all PIs are avoidable, and some may occur despite a patient specific prevention plan based on a patient's clinical condition and risks with implementation of appropriate interventions.[19,20] Development of a PI is dependent on both intrinsic and extrinsic factors.[19–22] Some of the intrinsic and extrinsic factors leading to unavoidable PIs in critical care patients include impaired tissue oxygenation, hypovolemia, body edema or anasarca, body habitus, hepatic dysfunction, peripheral vascular disease, chronic kidney disease, sensory impairment, altered levels of consciousness, age, end-of-life status, critical illness or injury, prone positioning, head-of-bed elevation,

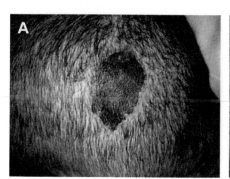 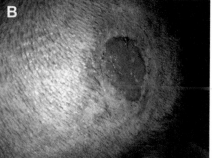

Fig. 15. Unstageable PI in ICU patient, occiput. (*A*) Prior to debridement. (*B*) Post–conservative sharp débridement. Wound healed by secondary intention.

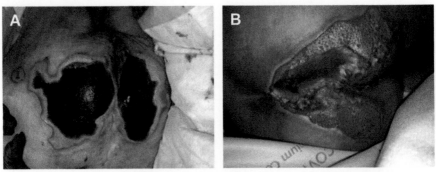

Fig. 16. Unstageable PI in ICU patient, buttocks. (*A*) Prior to debridement. (*B*) Post–conservative sharp débridement. Final outcome unknown.

vasopressor use, nutrition, hospital length of stay, use of medical devices, and behavioral risk factors.[20] These factors additionally may lead to delayed or compromised wound healing.

Palliative and Comfort-based/End-of-Life Care

For patients receiving palliative and comfort-based care, goals may transition to comfort and pain control rather than healing. Symptoms, such as odor and exudate control, infection prevention, and pain control, should be managed in patients at end of life.[13] These patients often require more frequent nursing care, such as turning to protect their skin, assistance with pain control, and incontinence care, to help prevent skin breakdown and contamination of wounds with urine and stool.[13]

Research Outcomes

Although there is a considerable amount of research around the prevention of PIs, research in the outcomes of unstageable PIs, including prevalence and incidence, in ICUs is lacking. A literature review revealed few research articles on critical care patients and unstageable PIs. One retrospective analysis of patients at a large academic medical center noted that 19 in a sample of 292 PIs presented as unstageable, with some patients found to have multiple PIs.[23] The article, however, did not indicate if the patients were located in an ICU. In a study associating Braden subscale scores

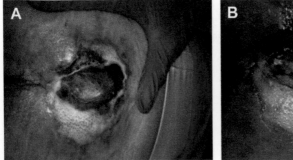
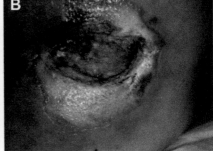

Fig. 17. Unstageable PI in ICU patient, sacrum. (*A*) Prior to debridement. (*B*) Post surgical débridement. Final outcome unknown.

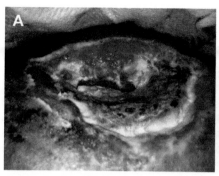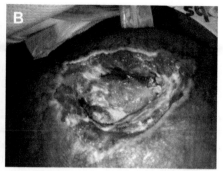

Fig. 18. Unstageable PI in ICU patient, ischium. (*A*) Prior to debridement. (*B*) Post–conservative sharp débridement. Final outcome unknown.

with PI risks in critical care patients presenting with stage 2 or greater PIs, 18 of 214 were noted to have unstageable PIs.[18] Results from another retrospective study found 47 of 78 patients with stage 2, stage 3, stage 4, or unstageable PIs were admitted to ICUs.[24] Three of the 78 patients included in that study developed unstageable PIs; however, it was unclear if the 3 patients with unstageable PIs were located in ICUs.[24] In a study of patients admitted to an ICU over a 7-year period at a Turkish university hospital, 15 patients (n = 359) were noted to have unstageable PIs, none of which healed.[25] One prospective case study of patients with advanced illness referred for palliative care reported that no patients with unstageable PIs (55 of 823 wounds) achieved complete healing.[26]

In the professional experience of the authors of this article, unstageable PIs that occur in critical care patients show a wide variety of outcomes (**Figs. 6–18**). Although some patients may go on to complete healing without surgical intervention, others require musculocutaneous flaps, and a smaller number may live with these wounds chronically.

SUMMARY

Although unstageable PIs likely always have existed, their identification and treatment have only begun to be more formally studied in recent years due to definition refinement of these wounds beginning in 2007. Correct identification of unstageable PIs proves challenging for health care providers and treatments vary. Key to the healing of these wounds in general, however, is débridement, when appropriate. This removal of nonviable tissue can be accomplished in multiple ways. Understanding the many types of débridement as well as their indications enhance clinical care. Although advancements in the science of unstageable PIs have been made, there is still much that is not known regarding the healing trajectories of these wounds and their outcomes in the critical care setting. Further research is warranted to improve identification, treatment, and outcomes.

DISCLOSURE

The authors have nothing to disclose.

REFERENCES

1. European Pressure Ulcer Advisory Panel, National Pressure Injury Advisory Panel, Pan Pacific Pressure Injury Alliance. Prevention and treatment of pressure

ulcers/injuries: clinical practice guideline. The International Guideline. In: Haesler E, editor. EPUAP/NPIAP/PPPIA; 2019. Available at: https://internationalguideline.com/static/pdfs/Quick_Reference_Guide-10Mar2019.pdf.

2. Edsberg L, Black J, Goldberg M, et al. Revised National Pressure Ulcer Advisory Panel pressure injury staging system: revised pressure injury staging system. J Wound Ostomy Continence Nurs 2016;43(6):585–97.

3. Charcot JM. Disorders of nutrition consecutive on lesions of the spinal cord and brain. In: Lectures on the diseases of the nervous system, delivered at La Salpetriere, vol. 1. London: The New Syndenham Society; 1877.

4. Pieper B, with the National Pressure ulcer Advisory Panel (NPUAP), editors. Pressure ulcers: prevalence, incidence, and implications for the future. Washington, DC: NPUAP; 2012.

5. Black J, Baharestani M, Cuddigan J, et al. National Pressure Ulcer Advisory Panel's updated pressure ulcer staging system. Urol Nurs 2007;27(2):144–50.

6. Zaratkiewicz S, Whitney J, Baker M, et al. Defining unstageable pressure ulcers as full-thickness wounds: are these wounds being misclassified? J Wound Ostomy Continence Nurs 2015;42(6):583–8.

7. Agrawal K, Chauhan N. Pressure ulcers: back to the basics. Indian J Plat Surg 2012;45(2):244–54.

8. Zaratkiewicz S. Defining unstageable pressure ulcers as full thickness wounds: is this definition consistent with clinical outcomes [dissertation]. Seattle (WA): University of Washington; 2015.

9. Lee YJ, Kim JY, Korean Association of Wound Ostomy Continence Nurses. Effects of pressure ulcer classification system education programme on knowledge and visual differential diagnostic ability of pressure ulcer classification and incontinence-associated dermatitis for clinical nurses in Korea. Int Wound J 2016;13(Suppl 1):26–32.

10. Alvey B, Hennen N, Heard H. Improving accuracy of pressure ulcer staging and documentation using a computerized clinical decision support system. J Wound Ostomy Continence Nurs 2012;39(6):607–12.

11. Suen W, Parker V, Harney L, et al. Internal medicine interns' and residents' pressure ulcer prevention and assessment attitudes and abilities: results of an exploratory study. Ostomy Wound Management 2012;58(4):28–35.

12. Levine J, Ayello E, Zulkowski K, et al. Pressure ulcer knowledge in medical residents: an opportunity for improvement. Adv Skin Wound Care 2012;25(3):115–7.

13. Bryant R, Nix D. Acute & chronic wounds: current management concepts. 5th edition. St Louis (MO): Elsevier; 2016.

14. Atkin L, Bucko Z, Conde M, et al. Implementing TIMERS: the race against hard-to-heal wounds. J Wound Care 2019;28(Suppl 3):S1–S49.

15. Doughty D, McNichol L. Wound, ostomy, and continence nurses Society core curriculum: wound management. 1st edition. Philadelphia: Wolters Kluwer; 2016.

16. Wound Ostomy and Continence Nurses Society. Guideline for prevention and management of pressure ulcers (injuries). In: WOCN clinical practice guideline series 2. Mt Laurel (NJ): Author; 2016. p. 97–8.

17. Carmel J, Colwell J, Goldberg M. Wound, ostomy and continent Society™ core curriculum: ostomy management. 1st edition. Philadelphia: Wolsters Kluwer; 2016.

18. Alderden J, Cummins MR, Pepper GA, et al. Midrange Braden subscale scores are associated with increased risk for pressure injury development among critical care patients. J Wound Ostomy Continence Nurs 2017;44(5):420–8.

19. Alvarez OM, Brindle CT, Langemo D, et al. The VCU pressure ulcer summit. J Wound Ostomy Continence Nurs 2016;43(5):1–9.
20. Edsberg LE, Langemo D, Baharestani MM, et al. Unavoidable pressure injury. J Wound Ostomy Continence Nurs 2014;4(4):313–34.
21. Black J, Edsberg L, Baharestani M, et al. Pressure ulcers: avoidable or unavoidable? Results of the National Pressure Ulcer Advisory Panel consensus conference. Ostomy Wound Manage 2011;57(2):24–37.
22. Schmitt S, Andries MK, Ashmore PM, et al. WOCN Society Position Paper: avoidable vs unavoidable pressure ulcers/injuries. J Wound Ostomy Continence Nurs 2017;44(5):458–68.
23. Backman C, Vanderloo SE, Miller TB, et al. Comparing physical assessment with administrative data for detecting pressure ulcers in a large Canadian academic health sciences centre. BMJ Open 2016;6(10):e012490.
24. Karahan A, Abbasoglu A, Isik S, et al. Factors affecting wound healing in individuals with pressure ulcers: a retrospective study. Ostomy Wound Management 2018;64(2):32–9.
25. Alcan AO, Giersbergen MV, Dincarslan G, et al. Healing status of pressure injuries among critically ill patients in a Turkish hospital: a descriptive, retrospective study. Wound Management Prev 2019;65(10):30–6.
26. Maida V, Ennis M, Corban J. Wound outcomes in patients with advanced illness. Int Wound J 2012;9(6):683–92.

Deep Tissue Pressure Injuries

Identification, Treatment, and Outcomes Among Critical Care Patients

Joyce M. Black, PhD, RN[a],*,
Christine T. Berke, MSN APRN-NP CWOCN-AP[b]

KEYWORDS

- Deep tissue pressure injury • Intensive care unit • Critical care nursing

KEY POINTS

- Critically Ill people are at high risk for developing deep tissue pressure injuries (DTPIs).
- DTPI frequently results in full-thickness ulceration.
- Progression of DTPI to ulceration can be rapid.
- DTPI in the critically ill patient can be life threatening.

DEEP TISSUE PRESSURE INJURY

Pressure injuries, or pressure ulcers, occur frequently in the critically ill patient. Deep tissue pressure injuries (DTPIs) are the most common type of pressure injury and seemingly occur suddenly and rapidly evolve into full-thickness pressure injury. This article addresses the pathophysiologic process that leads to DTPI and other conditions in the skin and soft tissue that can be misidentified as DTPI.

DEFINITION AND PRESENTATION OF DEEP TISSUE PRESSURE INJURY

The National Pressure Injury Advisory Panel (NPIAP) has defined DTPI as "Intact or non-intact skin with a localized area of persistent non-blanchable deep red, maroon, purple discoloration or epidermal separation revealing a dark wound bed or blood-filled blister. Pain and temperature change often precede skin color changes. Discoloration may appear differently in darkly pigmented skin. This injury results from intense

[a] College of Nursing, University of Nebraska Medical Center, Omaha, NE 68198-5330, USA;
[b] Center for Wound Healing and Ostomy Care, Nebraska Medicine, Omaha, NE 68198-1201, USA
* Corresponding author.
E-mail address: jblack@unmc.edu

Crit Care Nurs Clin N Am 32 (2020) 563–572
https://doi.org/10.1016/j.cnc.2020.08.006
0899-5885/20/© 2020 Elsevier Inc. All rights reserved.

and/or prolonged pressure and shear forces at the bone-muscle interface. The wound may evolve rapidly to reveal the actual extent of tissue injury or may resolve without tissue loss. If necrotic tissue, subcutaneous tissue, granulation tissue, fascia, muscle or other underlying structures are visible, this indicates a full thickness pressure injury (Unstageable, Stage 3 or Stage 4). Do not use DTPI to describe vascular, traumatic, neuropathic, or dermatologic conditions."[1] (**Fig. 1**).

RISK AND PREVALENCE OF PRESSURE INJURY IN THE CRITICALLY ILL

People who experience episodes of critical illness requiring care in intensive care units (ICUs) are at increased risk of developing pressure injuries in general, specifically DTPIs. Treatments associated with ICU level of care may include multiple invasive modalities (eg, mechanical ventilation, extracorporeal membrane oxygenation, hemodialysis, vasopressor agents, intra-aortic balloon pump, and ventricular assist devices). These treatments along with quickly changing clinical parameters (eg, blood pressure fluctuations, respiratory and circulatory status changes, altered mental status, and multiorgan or systems dysfunction) can contribute to prolonged episodes of impaired mobility and physical inactivity; decreased sensory perception and mental awareness;

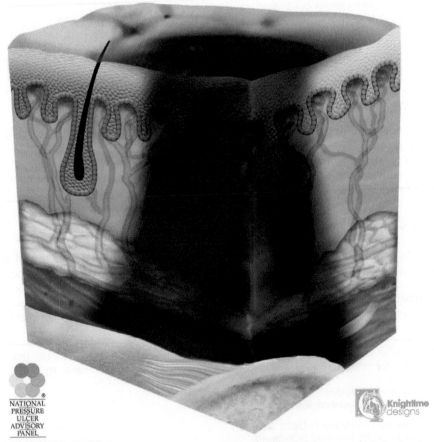

Fig. 1. Artist rendition of a DTPI (NPIAP). (©2016 National Pressure Ulcer Advisory Panel.)

limited or suboptimal nutritional intake; exposure to excesses in moisture from incontinence; emesis and/or drainage from lines, drives, airways, or wounds; decreased perfusion and oxygenation of tissues already under increased levels of pressure; and shear and friction forces. All of these are risk factors for the development of pressure injury. The higher rate of pressure injury development in the ICU is related to the higher level of disease and illness burden in this population. The risk factors for critically ill people are like any other population with the addition of the higher or intensified level of illness. The development of a pressure injury or DTPI in this population increases the threat for an additional comorbid and potentially life-threatening situation on top of an already severely compromised person.[2]

Studies have been conducted and published on the prevalence and/or incidence of pressure injuries in the ICU population. The reported results vary considerably and range from 13.1% to 45.5%.[2–4]

It is important to remember that prevalence is the number of existing cases identified on the day of the skin surveillance activity, whereas the incidence is the number of new cases that occur over a specific period of time determined by detailed observational parameters. It is important when reviewing published data to make sure personal/facility results are compared with the correct corresponding published rates.

THE NATURAL HISTORY OF DEEP TISSUE PRESSURE INJURY

One of the most unique aspects of DTPI is that the change in skin color from normal for the patient to purple or ecchymotic occurs rapidly. In many cases, the skin assessment done at the time of admission indicates no impairments of the skin, and, within 48 hours, the skin is described as "purple," "maroon," "bruised," or "ecchymotic," when there has been no documented trauma to the tissues during the intervening hours. **Fig. 2** depicts a DTPI in a patient who underwent coronary artery bypass 48 hours prior and when admitted to the ICU after surgery, her skin was intact. **Fig. 3** also illustrates a DTPI, but this patient was admitted to the hospital for acute-onset respiratory difficulty, placed on noninvasive ventilation, and placed in a 45° elevation of the head of the bed. The change in the skin was present 24 hours after admission.

PATHOPHYSIOLOGY OF DEEP TISSUE PRESSURE INJURY

DTPI derived its name from the fact that the injury occurs in the muscle rather than the skin. The cases presented in **Figs. 1** and **2** did not follow the learned material of pressure ulcers that has long stated that pressure ulcers start in the skin as a stage 1 and then progress to a full-thickness wound over several weeks in patients who are demented, bedridden, incontinent, and/or malnourished. For many years, if wounds were seen on the buttocks of patients who had been in surgery, the patterns of tissue damage were described as "cautery burns." For patients who were found down at scene, diagnoses such as soft tissue necrosis or rhabdomyolysis, were made. The pattern of DTPI from exposure to pressure, however, was increasingly clear, and early bench research explained what clinicians were seeing in the units. Some of the earliest bench research on the formation and pathogenesis of deep tissue injury (DTI) was done and is well explained by Oomens and colleagues.[5] This section is a summary of their work; the reader is referred to the work by Oomens for more in-depth explanation. To understand how DTPI develops quickly and evolves quickly, Oomens and colleagues[5] designed a series of experiments to examine cells placed under strain. When tissue is deformed by slow and moderate pressure, blood vessels are occluded, and the tissues become ischemic and acidotic and eventually die. This

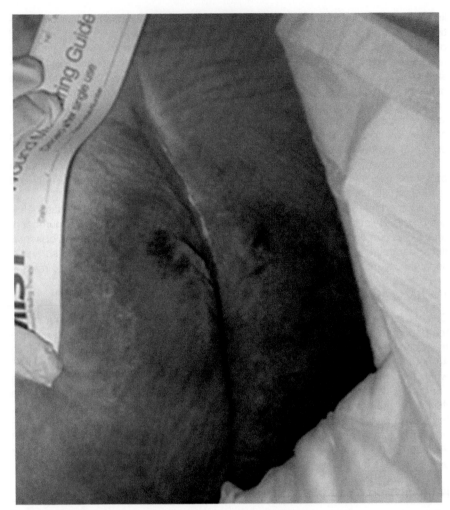

Fig. 2. DTPI 48 hours post–coronary artery bypass procedure.

model of pressure injury development is what was believed to lead to stage 1 pressure injury. When the intensity of the pressure is increased, the muscle cell membrane is destroyed, and the cell is very quickly damaged. The intense strain over a much shorter time frame leads to DTPI.

Of course, "How long does it take?" is a big question to scientists and clinicians. Several authors have focused on determining an injury threshold specific to muscle tissue in relation to DTPI development.[6–8] Linder-Ganz and colleagues[6] reported that muscle cell death occurred in an animal model subjected to 260 mm Hg to 525 mm Hg for 15 minutes to 1 hour or in muscles with 68 mm Hg applied pressure for more than 2 hours, indicating that magnitude of pressure is an important factor in muscle cell death. Although exact time frames cannot be identified, the greater the magnitude of pressure, the shorter the time frame to cell injury and death.

Shear force within the layers of tissue also occurs and contributes to tissue damage. Muscle cells are the most sensitive tissue to the effect of shear due to their

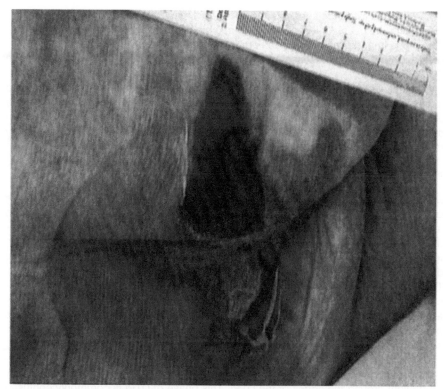

Fig. 3. DTPI 72 hours post–episode of acute respiratory distress (note the blistering).

arrangement in bundles and are the most sensitive to ischemia due to their high metabolic rate.[9] Recently, the impact of DTPI in adipose tissue also has been described.[10]

In more recent years, the idea of ischemic injury also has been cited as a cause of DTPI and is more familiar to the critical care clinician as the cause of pressure ulcers. But can ischemia alone lead to a DTPI, damaging the muscle cells? Ischemia as a result of sustained deformation of soft tissues leads to hypoxia, reduced nutrient supply, and impaired removal of metabolic waste products. Deprivation of nutrients and decrease in the pH level toward a more acidic extracellular environment due to accumulation of waste products eventually leads to cell death and tissue damage.[11]

The time that cells and tissues can endure ischemia without irreversible damage differs for the various tissues that potentially are involved in pressure injuries (eg, muscle, fat, and skin). Less intense deformations of tissues can lead to ischemia. Skeletal muscle tissues are not able to survive during ischemia lasting more than 6 hours. In animal experiments, the first signs of ischemic damage are found in skeletal muscle after 2 hours to 4 hours of sustained deformation.[12]

The clinical staff in critical care are well familiar with the problem of reperfusion injury seen after ischemic injuries, such as myocardial infarction, burns, and stroke. The same process occurs in DTPI; the reperfusion of blood into ischemic tissue causes cellular edema, tissue damage, and overproduction of reactive oxygen species, which may injure the endoplasmic reticulum. An inflammatory response is incited, and a mass of inflammatory mediators is released in the ischemic tissue which, in turn, results in the overproduction of cytotoxic oxygen-derived free radicals.[12]

Overall, this evidence suggests that DTPI as a result of mechanical loading occurs due to a combination of ischemia, lymphatic blockage, reperfusion and cell deformation.[13] It is important that clinicians are aware of the etiology of DTPI, in order to understand that a visual assessment alone is not a reliable indicator of early detection of DTPI.[14]

Some clinicians question if all pressure injuries are a result of pressure applied to muscle cells; thus, do all pressure injuries begin as DTPI? The short answer is no, there are other ways to deform cells that do not include pressure applied to muscle. Pressure injury of the lip from an endotracheal tube is a good example of a pressure injury that does not begin at a muscle level.

PRESENTATION OF DEEP TISSUE PRESSURE INJURY

DTPI presents as purple or maroon intact skin over a body area exposed to intense pressure or prolonged pressure. The ecchymotic appearance commonly is confused as a posttraumatic bruise; however, examination of the patient's history does not identify trauma to that body area. History of exposure to pressure is present 48 hours prior, for example, if a patient may have been found down at the scene, transferred a long distance on a backboard, or been in surgery for several hours (usually over 3 hours). These findings in the history may not be easy to determine; not all emergency medicine providers record these data. The bedside clinician should inquire from the family about the events that preceded hospitalization. Ischemic or destroyed muscle tissue is painful, so, in almost all cases, the history identifies that the patient was unconscious, sedated, anesthetized, or paralyzed and, therefore, unaware of the pain.

Approximately 48 hours to 72 hours after the tissue is purple, the epidermis lifts (epidermolysis), revealing a bright red and purple or dark wound bed. Shreds of skin may be present around the edges of the DTPI. This phase of DTPI is commonly confused with skin tears. Again, however, there is no evidence of trauma to the area. Because of the thickness of the skin in darkly pigmented skin, those skin remnants remain for a longer period usually 48 hours.

The final appearance of DTPI is either a blood blister or eschar. At this point, the pressure injury should be staged as unstageable. The time for this evolution is between 7 days and 10 days in most patients.

Establishing the time frame about a history of exposure to pressure is important, recognizing that in some patients the event of immobility was prior to hospital admission and, therefore, the DTPI actually was evolving at the time of admission but not yet visible.

DIFFERENTIAL DIAGNOSIS OF DEEP TISSUE PRESSURE INJURY

There are many conditions that cause skin to become purple and/or rapidly develop eschar or gangrene. It is important to distinguish those problems from DTPI. DTPI appears in a patient with a history of pressure and or shear in the body part with the identified wound. The DTPI is palpable and painful (if the patient is able to sense pain), but other conditions also can be palpable and painful. Some of the differential diagnoses for DTPI are presented in **Fig. 4**. It is beyond the scope of this article to discuss all these conditions, but it is important to establish a timeline of possible pressure-related injury if DTPI is suspected (eg, episode of the patient being found down and/or extended immobility prior to admission; prolonged operation/time in the operating room [OR], usually more than 3 hours and/or with episodes of documented hypoperfusion; prone or other specific controlled/prolonged position while in the OR that corresponds to the discolored area; and documentation/reports of sitting

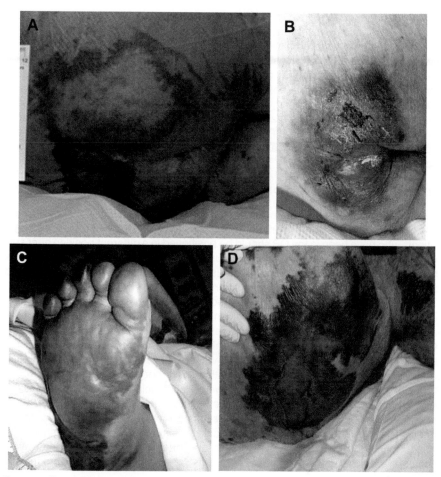

Fig. 4. Differential diagnosis of purple discoloration in skin and soft tissues. (*A*) Embolic shower after aortic clamp in OR. (*B*) Chronic friction injury. (*C*) Ischemia from vasopressors. (*D*) Hematoma post–pelvic fracture.

semirecumbent most of the day and/or night [head of bed elevated >45°, recliner or geriatric chair]). Knowing the history of the person's activity and the skin lesion/wound cannot be stressed enough; do not rely strictly on skin and wound examination for diagnosis of DTPI.[15,16]

DETERMINING PRESENCE ON ADMISSION

Because many DTPIs can begin prior to hospital admission, it is important to understand the current reporting structure to Centers for Medicaid & Medicare Services (CMS) via the *International Classification of Diseases, Tenth Revision* codes. Hospitals can classify DTPI that were evolving at the time of admission as "present on admission" (POA). The CMS do not have a mandatory time frame for determining if a condition is POA. Many hospitals have created policy that skin assessment be performed within 4 hours and that any condition considered POA be identified in 24 hours. Although this policy is excellent clinical practice, these time frames do not exist within the CMS recording structure. DTPI tends to be the condition that is missed as a POA condition. If a patient was exposed to intense pressure that damaged muscle cells less than 48 hours from admission, the skin likely is normal on admission. Then, several hours later, the skin turns purple. So, the color change developing later leads clinicians to believe that the DTPI occurred during the hospital stay. A thorough history helps determine if there was exposure to pressure prior to admission in the body areas now seen as purple. At that point, a decision can be made if this DTPI had begun prior to admission and can be coded as POA. There are outliers to the 48-hour time frame from exposure to pressure to the visible purple skin, but not many. Patients who are obese tend to have a delayed presentation. DTPI on anterior body surfaces often appears within 24 hours.

PREVENTION AND TREATMENT OF DEEP TISSUE PRESSURE INJURY

The prevention and treatment of patients at high risk for developing DTPI must include consistent off-loading of a high-risk/affected area; this cannot be stressed enough. Patients who have been in the OR should be positioned in a different position after surgery than was used for any recent/previous surgery. Patients who require dialysis should be positioned off the affected site (supine or side lying positions may need to be considered, depending on the location of the DTPI).[2]

For those persons in ICU who are deemed unstable for regular turning and repositioning, small frequent shifts in body position can be made. Staff need to assess a patient's tolerance to these smaller incremental shifts and gradually increase to a standard level of repositioning (eg, 30° lateral positioning every 30 minutes to 2 hours), allowing at least 10 minutes for the patient's vital signs to equilibrate before attempting additional repositioning maneuvers. If a patient does not tolerate incremental turns, strategies can be considered that include weight shifts (hips and shoulders), passive range of motion, repositioning of extremities, head rotation, heel elevation/floating, and lower-angle (less than 30°) turns. Because of the often rapid changes in a patient's condition in the ICU, turning and repositioning (regular or incremental) should be based individually on a patient's response and attempted more often than every 2 hours. Removing pressure from damaged tissue aids in its recovery through the restoration of blood flow.[2]

When a DTPI has been identified, soft multilayer silicone foam dressings[2,17,18] and air-fluidized beds[19] have been shown to reduce the evolution and ulceration extent of the DTPI. Both of these therapies likely reduce the severity of the injury by reducing pressure and shear in the area of the DTPI.

In a longitudinal prospective historical case-control study (N = 60), Honaker and colleagues[20] showed that the addition of noncontact low-frequency ultrasound, within 5 days of onset, reduced the severity of DTPI, its total surface area, and its final pressure injury stage. The surface area of the DTPI in the treatment group decreased by a mean of 8.8 cm^2 compared with a mean decrease in the control group of only 0.3 cm^2. In this study, 57% of the DTPI treated with standard care became unstageable compared with 3% of the group treated with noncontact low-frequency ultrasound.

OUTCOMES

Outcomes of DTPI can be devastating and life altering (as well as limb threatening), if the injury is not detected early and/or not treated aggressively.[20] In the case series by Berke and Black,[21] few of the DTPIs healed (10%), and healing versus nonhealing was correlated to the age of the patient ($P<.05$) and relative immobility ($P<.05$). Débridement was done in 55% of the cases, but few (5%) underwent closure with a flap.

Sepsis from the DTPI occurred in 28% of patients, and 21% of the patients died as a result of the DTPI. Diabetes and peripheral vascular disease were correlated with sepsis ($P<.007$ and $P<0.000$, respectively). In a multivariate model, DTPI of the sacrum increased the risk of sepsis ($P<.003$). DTPI of the heel required amputation in 13%, and amputation was more likely in patients with diabetes ($P<.000$) and peripheral vascular disease ($P<.05$). Children with DTPI seem to resolve the injuries more rapidly and with less tissue loss than in adults; the reason for this difference is not understood.

SUMMARY

DTPI is a dangerous form of pressure injury due to delay between exposure to pressure and the appearance of discolored skin. Furthermore, by the time discolored skin is evident, the damage is done to the muscle. Complete off-loading and ultrasonic mist are the best options for treatment. Both interventions reduce ongoing ischemia in the tissue. Débridement often is needed for resolution of the wound. Unfortunately, sepsis, diverting colostomy, and amputation often are required.

DISCLOSURE

J.M. Black is a Consultant for Mölnlycke Health Care, Wound Vision, Hill-Rom, and Sage Products: A Division of Stryker Medical and Acelity. She is a member of the Speakers' Bureau for Mölnlycke Health Care, Wound Vision, Hill-Rom, and Sage Products: A Division of Stryker Medical and Acelity. C.T. Berke has nothing to disclose.

REFERENCES

1. Edsberg LE, Black JM, Goldberg M, et al. Revised national pressure ulcer advisory panel pressure injury staging system: revised pressure injury staging system. J Wound Ostomy Continence Nurs 2016;43(6):585–97.
2. European Pressure Ulcer Advisory Panel, National Pressure Injury Advisory Panel and Pan Pacific Pressure Injury Alliance. In: Haesler E, editor. Prevention and treatment of pressure ulcers/injuries: clinical practice guideline. The International guideline. Boston, MA: EPUAP/NPIAP/PPPIA; 2019. p. 28–9.
3. He M, Tang A, Ge X, et al. Pressure ulcers in the intensive care unit: an analysis of skin barrier risk factors. Adv Skin Wound Care 2016;29(11):493–8.
4. Amirah MFY, Rasheed AMY, Parameaswari PJ, et al. Pressure injury prevalence and risk factors among adults at a large intensive care unit. J Intensive Crit Care 2019;5(2):1–9.
5. Oomens CWJ, Bader DL, Loerakker S, et al. Pressure indicated deep tissue injury explained. Ann Biomed Eng 2014;43:297–305.
6. Linder-Ganz E, Engelberg S, Scheinowitz M, et al. Pressure-time cell death threshold for albino rat skeletal muscles as related to pressure sore biomechanics. J Biomech 2006;39(14):2725–32.
7. Stekelenburg A, Strijkers GJ, Parusel H, et al. Role of ischemia and deformation in the onset of compression-induced deep tissue injury: MRI-based studies in a rat model. J Appl Physiol 2007;102(5):2002–11.
8. Gefen A, van Nierop B, Bader DL, et al. Strain-time cell death threshold for skeletal muscle in a tissue-engineered model system for deep tissue injury. J Biomech 2008;41(9):2003–12.
9. Gefen A, Gefen N, Linder-Ganz E, et al. In vivo muscle stiffening under bone compression promotes deep pressure sores. J Biomech Eng 2005;127:512–24.

10. Edsberg L, Call E, Black J. Histology of deep tissue pressure injury: what can be learned from cadavers. In: National pressure ulcer advisory panel conference, Las Vegas, NV; 2018.

11. Loerakker S, Manders E, Strijkers GJ, et al. The effects of deformation, ischemia, and reperfusion on the development of muscle damage during prolonged loading. J Appl Physiol 2011;111(4):1168–77.

12. Jiang L, Tu Q, Wang Y, et al. Ischeumia-reperfusion injury-induced histological changes affecting early stage pressure ulcer development in a rat model. Ostomy Wound Manage 2011;57(2):55–60.

13. Peart J. The aetiology of deep tissue injury: a literature review. Br J Nurs 2016; 25(15):840–3.

14. Berlowitz D, Brienza D. Are all pressure ulcers the result of deep tissue injury? A review of the literature. Ostomy Wound Manage 2007;53(10):34–8.

15. Black JM, Brindle CT, Honaker JS. Differential diagnosis of suspected deep tissue injury. Int Wound J 2015;13(4):531–9.

16. Berke CT. Pathology and clinical presentation of friction injuries: case series and literature review. J Wound Ostomy Continence Nurs 2015;42(1):47–61.

17. Sullivan RA. Two-year retrospective review of suspected deep tissue injury evolution in adult acute care patients. Ostomy Wound Manage 2013;59(9):30–9.

18. Sullivan R. Use of a soft silicone foam dressing to change the trajectory of destruction associated with suspected deep tissue pressure ulcers. Medsurg Nurs J 2015;24:237–67.

19. Allen L, McGarrah B, Barrett D, et al. Air-fluidized therapy in patients with suspected deep tissue injury: a case series. J Wound Ostomy Continence Nurs 2012;39:555–61.

20. Honaker JS, Forston MR, Davis EA, et al. The effect of adjunctive noncontact low frequency ultrasound on deep tissue pressure injury. Wound Repair Regen 2016; 24(6):1081–8.

21. Berke CT, Black J. Retrospective study to identify a risk profile for pressure related deep tissue injury. In: Poster presentation. National Wound Ostomy Continence Nurse Conference, Salt Lake City (UT); June 9, 2007.

Pressure Injuries Among Critical Care Patients

Nancy Munoz, DCN, MHA, RDN, LD, FAND[a,b,]*

KEYWORDS

- Nutrition • Pressure injury • Protein • Macronutrients • Micronutrients
- International guideline • Nutrients

KEY POINTS

- Nutrition is an important component in the prevention and treatment of pressure injuries.
- Although the point at which insufficient nutrient consumption affects the body's capability to support skin integrity has not been demarcated, what is known is that reduced intake of food and fluids/water and weight loss can increase the risk of developing pressure injuries.
- Protein and its building blocks, amino acids, are essential for tissue growth and repair during all phases of wound healing.
- Sufficient macronutrients (carbohydrates, protein, fats, and water) and micronutrients (vitamins and minerals) are vital for the body to support tissue integrity and prevent breakdown.

INTRODUCTION

Nutrition is an important component in the prevention and treatment of pressure injuries (PIs). Nutrients are required in the right amount by each body organ system to support growth, development, maintenance, and repair of body tissues. The National Pressure Injury Advisory Panel (NPIAP) defines PIs as "a localized damage to the skin and/or underlying soft tissue usually over a bony prominence or related to a medical or other device. The injury can present as intact skin or an open ulcer and may be painful. The injury occurs as a result of intense and/or prolonged pressure or pressure in combination with shear. The tolerance of soft tissue for pressure and shear may also be affected by microclimate, nutrition, perfusion, co-morbidities and condition of the soft tissue."[1] Nutrition is a confounding factor in the development of PIs. Nutritional deprivation and inadequate dietary intake are risk factors for the development of PIs and impaired wound healing.

[a] UMass Amherst, Amherst, MA, USA; [b] Nutrition and Foodservice, VA Southern Nevada Healthcare System, 7041 Solana Ridge Drive, North Las Vegas, NV 89084, USA
* UMass Amherst, Amherst, MA.
E-mail address: Dr.NMunozRD@outlook.com

Crit Care Nurs Clin N Am 32 (2020) 573–587
https://doi.org/10.1016/j.cnc.2020.08.007
0899-5885/20/© 2020 Elsevier Inc. All rights reserved.

ccnursing.theclinics.com

Pls are a costly condition that have a significant impact on patient morbidity, mortality, and quality of life. The incidence and prevalence of Pls is high in all health care settings. The International Pressure Ulcer Prevalence Survey, 2006 to 2015, reports the prevalence of Pls in the United States as follows[2]:

- Overall PI prevalence in the United States: 9.3% in 2015
- In-house acquired PI: 3.1%–3.4% in 2013 to 2015
- Facility-acquired prevalence in acute care: 2.9% in 2015
- Long-term acute care: 28.8% in 2015
- Long-term care in house acquired: 5.4% in 2015

Each year, more than 2.5 million people in the United States develop Pls. In 2019, $26.8 billion dollars were spent in treating Pls.[3]

NUTRITION AND RISK FOR DEVELOPING PRESSURE INJURIES

Research suggests that there is a moderate statistical link between the nutritional status of individuals and the development of Pls.[4] The European Pressure Ulcer Advisory Panel (NPIAP) Pan Pacific Pressure Injury Alliance (PPPIA) Clinical Practice Guideline (International 2019 CPG) outlines that 40% (out of 50 studies reviewed) identify nutrition variables as a significant predictor of PI development.[4]

Nutrition risk factors associated with PI development include malnutrition, unintended weight loss, low body mass index (BMI), increased nutrient needs, inadequate food and fluid intake, and syndromes, such as sarcopenia, sarcopenic obesity, and cachexia.

Malnutrition

Defined as "a state resulting from lack of intake or uptake of nutrition that leads to altered body composition (decreased fat free mass) and body cell mass leading to diminished physical and mental function and impaired clinical outcome from disease," malnutrition covers several nutrition disorders that encompass undernutrition, wasting, vitamin and mineral deficiency, obesity, and malnutrition that occur as a result of the presence of chronic diseases.[5,6] Several organizations have outlined criteria to be utilized in diagnosing malnutrition. **Table 1** outlines the diagnostic criteria set forth by the American Society for Parenteral and Enteral Nutrition (ASPEN)/Academy of Nutrition and Dietetics, European Society of Clinical Nutrition and Metabolism (ESPEN), and the Global Leadership Initiative (GLIM).

Prevalence of Malnutrition

Malnutrition causes more ill health worldwide than any other health condition.[6] Globally, overweight and obesity in adults are at record high levels, with 38.9% of adults being overweight or obese.[6] Universally, malnutrition affects 30% to 50% of all hospitalized patients.[7] For decades, the presence of malnutrition has been linked to undesirable clinical, functional, and economic outcomes. The presence of malnutrition can contribute to increased risk for comorbidities, added hospital length of stay (LOS), and greater readmission rate, health care costs, and mortality.[8] A study of Medicare beneficiaries aged greater than or equal to 65 years reported that 75% of their study participants were malnourished. In the United States, the cost of malnutrition and associated comorbidities is estimated to be more than $15.5 billion per year.[9]

Table 1
Criteria to diagnose malnutrition

	American Society for Parenteral and Enteral Nutrition/ Academy of Nutrition and Dietetics	European Society of Clinical Nutrition and Metabolism	Global Leadership Initiative
Unintended weight loss	X		X
Low BMI		X	X
Loss of muscle mass	X		X
Loss of subcutaneous fat	X	X	
Localized or generalized fluid accumulation	X		
Decreased functional status	X		
Reduced food intake or assimilation	X		X
Disease burden/inflammation			X
A risk per validated screening tool		X	
	Two of the 6 characteristics must be present	Once the person is deemed at risk by a validated screening tool, 1 of the other 2 characteristics must be present.	One phenotype and 1 etiologic characteristic must be present

Data from White JV, Guenter P, Jensen G, et al. Consensus statement: Academy of Nutrition and Dietetics and American Society for Parenteral and Enteral Nutrition: characteristics recommended for the identification and documentation of adult malnutrition (undernutrition). J Parenter Enteral Nutr. 36(3):275–83; and Cederholm T, Jensen GL, Correia MITD, et al. GLIM criteria for the diagnosis of malnutrition - A consensus report from the global clinical nutrition community. Clin Nutr. 2019;38(1):1–9.

MALNUTRITION AND PRESSURE INJURIES

Although the point at which insufficient nutrient consumption affects the body's capability to support skin integrity has not been demarcated, what is known is that reduced intake of food and fluids/water and weight loss can increase the risk of developing PIs.[10] In individuals with PI, inadequate food and fluid intake can contribute to impaired wound healing rate.[11] Unplanned/involuntary weight loss is considered a main risk factor for both malnutrition and PI development.[12]

A form of malnutrition in which intake of nutrients is greater than the amount needed to support growth, development, and metabolism is called overnutrition. This can result in individuals becoming overweight or obese.

In the United States, the rate of obesity has reached to epidemic levels. In 2015 to 2016 the prevalence of obesity was reported as 39.8% of the US population.[13] Comorbidities associated with obesity include chronic conditions, such as diabetes, cardiovascular disease, hypertension, dyslipidemia, respiratory diseases, and impaired wound healing. The limited mobility frequently connected with obese individuals and struggle with self-repositioning can contribute further to the development of PI.[14]

WOUND HEALING PHASES AND NUTRITION

The wound healing process is a cascade of events consisting of 4 distinct and overlapping phases. Protein and its building blocks, amino acids, are essential for tissue growth and repair during all phases of wound healing. The inflammatory process, cell proliferation, and tissue granulation all require the availability of adequate amount of protein and amino acids in the right proportions.[15] **Table 2** describes the phases of wound healing and the key healing factors and nutrients.[16–18]

ROLE OF NUTRIENTS IN PRESSURE INJURY PREVENTION AND TREATMENT

Sufficient macronutrients (carbohydrates, protein, fats, and water) and micronutrients (vitamins and minerals) are vital for the body to support tissue integrity and prevent breakdown. The International 2019 CPG nutrition recommendations suggest providing 30 kcal/kg of body weight to 35 kcal/kg of body weight per day for adults with a PI who are malnourished or at risk of malnutrition. The recommendation for protein is 1.25 g/ kg of weight body per day to 1.5 g/ kg of body weight per day for adults with a PI who are malnourished or at risk of malnutrition.[4] Encouraging patients to consume adequate amount of kilocalories (energy) to support nutritional needs helps the body synthesize collagen and nitrogen in sufficient amount to spare protein from being utilized as an energy source. Aside from being the most concentrate source of calories, fat is essential to support cell membranes, and the immune system.

Because there is no precise research defining optimal caloric needs to prevent PIs, the International 2019 CPG suggest that energy and protein intake be optimized for each individual. This should be done within the context of the individual's nutritional status (eg, current, usual, and goal weights) and clinical condition.[4]

The International 2019 CPG provides specific direction on energy needs for individuals with a PI. See **Table 3** for a list of all the International 2019 CPG nutrition recommendations. **Table 4** describes the strength of the evidence and the strength of the evidence for each recommendation. Each recommendation includes a list of implementation consideration drafted and available in the International 2019 CPG document.[4]

As seen in **Table 4**, the International 2019 CPG provide specific caloric guidance for individuals with a PI. In the past 3 decades, several studies have directly and indirectly shown the importance of providing sufficient kilocalories and protein to patients with a PI. A study by Iizaka and colleagues reported[19] that providing adequate kilocalories and protein was associated with wound healing for deep PI.[19]

As discussed previously, protein is an important nutrient for all phases of wound healing. Protein plays an important role in protecting the immune system; synthesis of enzymes needed for cell replication and collagen synthesis. **Table 3** outlines International 2019 CPG nutrition recommendations for individuals at risk for or with an actual PI.

Since 1933, researchers have been reporting that increased protein levels promote positive patient outcomes in PI healing rates. Breslow and colleagues[20] reported that individuals consuming greater levels of protein and calories had statistically significant reduction in PI surface compared with those receiving a regular diet.

Water is the solvent for vitamins, minerals, glucose, and other nutrients. Water also is required to move nutrients through the body and to eliminate waste products. In healthy individuals, water/fluid intake should be approximately 30 mL/kg of body weight per day or 1 mL per kilocalorie consumed per day. Individuals with or at risk for dehydration, increased temperature, profuse sweating, and heavily exuding

Table 2
Phases of wound healing and key healing factors

Wound Healing Phase	Description	Key Healing Factors	Key Nutrients
Coagulation/hemostasis	The actual wounding and initiation of the healing process	Platelets, growth factors[a]	Protein: needed to release growth factors and to activate macrophages Calories are needed to spare protein for tissue build-up Vitamin A: improves cell mediated immunity B vitamins: cofactors in enzyme activity Vitamin K: needed for blood clotting Iron: optimizes tissue perfusion
Inflammatory	Cleaning phase	Neutrophils: white blood cells—essential component of immune system Macrophages: large phagocytic cells found in stationary form in the tissues or as a mobile white blood cell, especially at sites of infection Proteases: enzyme that breaks down proteins and peptide	Protein: main component of lymphocytes, leukocytes, and phagocytes Calories: needed to spare protein for tissue build-up Fats: source of calories, precursors for prostaglandins (which regulate numerous activities in cellular inflammation Vitamin C: monocyte movement into wound tissue → macrophages during inflammatory phase Vitamin A: necessary for wound débridement, immune cell formation, monocytes, and macrophages B vitamins: cofactors in enzyme activity Vitamin K: fibrin formation, blood clotting Copper: lymphocyte synthesis Iron: optimizes tissue perfusion Zinc: produces antibodies and activates lymphocytes

(continued on next page)

Table 2 *(continued)*			
Wound Healing Phase	Description	Key Healing Factors	Key Nutrients
Proliferative	Rebuilding phase	Macrophages Fibroblasts Endothelial cells Collagen	Protein: main component of lymphocytes, leukocytes, and phagocytes Calories needed to spare protein for tissue build-up Vitamin A: collagen synthesis, epithelialization Vitamin C: angiogenesis, collagen formation, fibroblast proliferation B vitamins: cofactors in enzyme activity Iron: optimizes tissue perfusion, collagen synthesis Zinc: needed for cells with rapid apoptosis/proliferative rate (inflammatory, epithelial, and fibroblast cells)
Maturation and remodeling	Strengthening, tensile strength increases	Collagen remodeling Capillary regression	Protein, vitamin C, vitamin A, zinc: needed for collagen synthesis Calories: needed to spare protein for tissue build-up B vitamins: cofactors in enzyme activity Iron: optimizes tissue perfusion

[a] Growth factor: a substance, such as a vitamin or hormone, which is required for the stimulation of growth in living cells.

Data from Refs.[16–18] and Munoz N, Posthauer ME, Cereda E, et al. Nutrition, essential for pressure injury prevention and healing: the 2019 international guideline recommendations. Submitted for publication, 2020.

Table 3 International guideline nutrition recommendations, 2019		
Number	**Recommendation**	**SoE; SoR or GPS**
1.10	Consider the impact of impaired nutritional status on the risk of PIs.	SoE = C; SoR = ↑
4.1	Conduct nutritional screening for individuals at risk of a PI.	SoE = B1; SoR = ↑↑
4.2	Conduct a comprehensive nutrition assessment for adults at risk of a PI who are screened to be at risk of malnutrition and for all adults with a PI.	SoE = B2; SoR = ↑↑
4.3	Develop and implement an individualized nutrition care plan for individuals with, or at risk of, a PI who are malnourished or who are at risk of malnutrition.	SoE = B2; SoR = ↑↑
4.4	Optimize energy intake for individuals at risk of PIs who are malnourished or at risk of malnutrition.	SoE = B2; SoR = ↑
4.5	Adjust protein intake for individuals at risk of PIs who are malnourished or at risk of malnutrition.	GPS
4.6	Provide 30–35 kcal/kg body weight/d for adults with a PI who are malnourished or at risk of malnutrition.	SoE = B1; SoR = ↑
4.7	Provide 1.25–1.5 g protein/kg body weight/d for adults with a PI who are malnourished or at risk of malnutrition.	SoE = B1; SoR = ↑↑
4.8	Offer high-calorie, high-protein fortified foods and/or nutritional supplements in addition to the usual diet for adults who are at risk of developing a PI and who are also malnourished or at risk of malnutrition, if nutritional requirements cannot be achieved by normal dietary intake.	SoE = C; SoR = ↑
4.9	Offer high-calorie, high-protein nutritional supplements in addition to the usual diet for adults with a PI who are malnourished or at risk of malnutrition, if nutritional requirements cannot be achieved by normal dietary intake.	SoE = B1; SoR = ↑↑
4.10	Provide high-calorie, high-protein, arginine, zinc and antioxidant oral nutritional supplements or enteral formula for adults with a category/stage II or greater PI who are malnourished or at risk of malnutrition.	SoE = B1; SoR = ↑
4.11	Discuss the benefits and harms of enteral or parenteral feeding to support overall health in light of preferences and goals of care with individuals at risk of PIs who cannot meet their nutritional requirements through oral intake despite nutritional interventions.	GPS

(continued on next page)

Table 3 *(continued)*		
Number	Recommendation	SoE; SoR or GPS
4.12	Discuss the benefits and harms of enteral or parenteral feeding to support PI treatment in light of preferences and goals of care for individuals with PIs who cannot meet their nutritional requirements through oral intake despite nutritional interventions.	SoE = B1; SoR = ↑
4.13	Provide and encourage adequate water/fluid intake for hydration for an individual injury, when compatible with goals of care and clinical conditions.	GPS
4.14	Conduct age-appropriate nutritional screening and assessment for neonates and children at risk of PIs.	GPS
4.15	For neonates and children with or at risk of PIs who have inadequate oral intake, consider fortified foods, age-appropriate nutritional supplements, or EN or PN support.	GPS
22.2	Provide PI education, skills training and psychosocial support to individuals with or at risk of PIs.	SoE = C; SoR = ↑

Abbreviations: GPS, Good Practice Statement; SOE, Strength of the Evidence; SOR, Strength of the Recommendation.

Adapted from European Pressure Ulcer Advisory Panel, National Pressure Injury Advisory Panel and Pan Pacific Pressure Injury Alliance. Prevention and Treatment of Pressure Ulcers/Injuries: Clinical Practice Guideline. The International Guideline. Emily Haesler (Ed.). EPUAP/NPIAP/PPPIA; 2019, with permission.

wounds should be provided with additional fluids. See **Table 3** for review of the International 2019 CPG fluid/water recommendations.

As seen in **Table 2**, several vitamins and minerals (micronutrients) play important roles in the treatment of PI. In the past, megadoses of vitamin and minerals had been prescribed for individuals with PI. The International 2019 CPG report that there is no evidence to support this practice. For individuals at risk for vitamin and mineral or with an actual deficiency, a multivitamin (MVI) should be prescribed.[4]

NUTRITION SCREENING

Nutritional screening be conducted on all individuals at risk of a PI (see **Table 3**).[4] Any member of the interprofessional team that has been trained and considered competent to use the screening tool can complete the nutrition screen.[21] The tool selected for use in health care facilities should be a validated instrument that is easy to use, economical, low risk for the individual being screened, and appropriate for determining nutritional risk in all types of people, to include individuals with fluid shifts and those in which weight and height cannot be obtained easily.[22,23] Within a health care facility, nutrition screening, and rescreening should be conducted in accordance with the mandates outlined by accrediting bodies and the facilities internal policies.

Frequently used validated nutritional screening instruments include Mini Nutritional Assessment (MNA), Malnutrition Universal Screening Tool (MUST), Nutrition Risk

Table 4 Strengths of evidence rating for recommendation	
Strengths of Evidence	
A	• More than 1 high-quality level I study providing direct evidence • Consistent body of evidence
B1	• Level 1 studies of moderate or low quality providing direct evidence • Level 2 studies of high or moderate quality providing direct evidence • Most studies have consistent outcomes and inconsistencies can be explained
B2	• Level 2 studies of low quality providing direct evidence • Level 3 or 4 studies (regardless of quality) providing direct evidence • Most studies have consistent outcomes and inconsistencies can be explained
C	• Level 5 studies (indirect evidence) for example, studies in normal human subjects, humans with other types of chronic wounds, animal models • A body of evidence with inconsistencies that cannot be explained, reflecting genuine uncertainty surrounding the topic
GPS	Good practice statement • Statements that are not supported by a body of evidence, as listed above, but considered by the GGG to be significant for clinical practice.
Strengths of Recommendation	
↑↑	Strong positive recommendation: definitely do it
↑	Weak positive recommendation: probably do it
↔	No specific recommendation
↓	Weak negative recommendation: probably do not do it
↓↓	Strong negative recommendation: definitely do not do it

Adapted from European Pressure Ulcer Advisory Panel, National Pressure Injury Advisory Panel and Pan Pacific Pressure Injury Alliance. Prevention and Treatment of Pressure Ulcers/Injuries: Clinical Practice Guideline. The International Guideline. Emily Haesler (Ed.). EPUAP/NPIAP/PPPIA; 2019, with permission.

Screening 2002 (NRS), and the Short Nutritional Assessment Questionnaire (SNAQ)[22–30] All these screening tools have been validated for identifying nutritional risk (**Table 5**).[31–37]

NUTRITION ASSESSMENT

After the screening process and referral to a registered dietitian nutritionist (RDN), a nutrition assessment is initiated for adults at risk of a PI who are screened to be at risk of malnutrition and for all adults with a PI (see **Table 3**).[4] The evaluation of an individual's nutritional status involves the interpretation of anthropometric, biochemical, clinical, and dietary facts.[21] Basic information included in a nutrition assessment for individuals at risk for development of skin impairment, including PIs includes[21]:

- Medical history, diagnosis, and recent changes in medical conditions
- Risk factors for development of or history of PIs
- Anthropometric measurements to include height, weight, weight history, and significant weight shifts
- Eating ability, level of assistance required, and chewing or swallowing difficulties
- Current food/fluid intake compared with estimated nutrition needs

Table 5
Summary of the nutrition screening tool validation studies

Nutrition Screening Tool	Evidence for Identifying Pressure Injury Risk Status	Evidence for Identifying Factors Associated with Pressure Injury Risk	Clinical Setting
MNA, full version[31]	Yes	Yes	Older adults in community settings[25] Older adults in long-term care[27] Older adults with PIs and multiple comorbidities[26] Older adults at nutritional risk in long term care and community settings[30] Older adults in acute care, long-term care and community settings[28]
MUST[32]	No	Yes	Older adults in acute care, long-term care and community settings[28]
NRS, 2002[33]	No	No	Adults in acute care[23] Older adults in acute care, long-term care and community settings[28]
SNAQ[34,35]	No	No	Adults in acute care[24] Older adults in residential care[24]
Seniors in the Community: Risk Evaluation for Eating and Nutrition (SCREEN)[36,37]	No	No	Older adults in community settings[36]

Adapted from European Pressure Ulcer Advisory Panel, National Pressure Injury Advisory Panel and Pan Pacific Pressure Injury Alliance. Prevention and Treatment of Pressure Ulcers/Injuries: Clinical Practice Guideline. The International Guideline. Emily Haesler (Ed.). EPUAP/NPIAP/PPPIA; 2019, with permission.

- Drug regime, including herbal supplements and over-the-counter medications that can have an effect on intake and food–medication interactions
- Food allergies, intolerances, or cultural food preferences
- Biochemical data—laboratory data and/or medical tests
- Food preferences
- Nutrition-focused physical examination

The nutrition assessment should be completed by an RDN with input from members of the interprofessional nutrition team. Research supports that the use of a comprehensive, interdisciplinary nutritional protocol can improve both PI wound healing rates and decrease hospital LOS while curtailing treatment cost.[38]

Laboratory values are a good indicator of the patent's overall health status. Laboratory tests, such as albumin and prealbumin, are not sensitive indicators of an individual's nutritional status.[39]

NUTRITION INTERVENTIONS

Based on the information collected in the nutrition assessment, the RDN defines interventions to help the individual meet their nutritional needs. As part of this process, the RDN calculates estimated needs for kilocalories, protein, and fluids and translate these calculations into foods and interventions for the individual to consume.

Basic nutrition interventions rely on a food-first approach and often focus on improving the individuals' intake. Approaches for improving oral intake include

- Nutritional counseling
- Providing fortified foods
- Liberalizing dietary restrictions (if these interfere with adequate intake)
- Providing assistance during meals
- Honoring cultural, religious food preferences
- Ensuring a pleasant eating environment

Nutrient-dense and fortified foods can provide the increased calories and protein needed without overwhelming the person with volume of food. Examples of fortified foods involve adding dry milk to cooked cereal, mashed potatoes or casseroles. Swapping Greek yogurt for regular yogurt also can help increase nutrient intake. Providing a homemade milkshake or a meat sandwich can be the perfect intervention for many individuals.

Patients suffering from chronic disease or at risk for developing PI often are unable to meet their nutritional needs. For these patients, the use of oral nutritional supplements (ONS) can be an effective strategy to help them meet their kilocalorie and protein needs. International 2019 CPG recommendations support the use of ONS with micronutrients for individuals with a PI who are malnourished (or at risk) (see **Table 3**).[4]

A systematic review of randomized controlled trials concluded that the use of ONS normally is a well-tolerated intervention. The use of ONS can result in both positive energy balance and clinical benefits, especially if ONS (1.5–2.4 kcal/mL) are consumed between meals.[40]

Research indicates that the provision of enteral nutrition (EN) or parenteral nutrition (PN) has limited impact on preventing PI for those at risk.[41–44] When used, the goal of artificial nutrition (whether EN or PN) is to improve the individuals nutritional status, promote healing and restore their immune function.[45,46] When PI healing has stalled and oral intake is inadequate to support the patient's nutritional needs, EN or PN should be considered, if it is in accordance with the individual's goal for care (see **Table 3**).

INDIVIDUALIZED CARE PLAN

Development and communication of an individualized care plan are the final steps of completing a comprehensive nutrition assessment. The International 2019 CPG propose the development and implementation of an individualized nutrition care plan for individuals with, or at risk of, a PI who are malnourished or who are at risk of malnutrition (see **Table 3**).

The care plan process is guided by both the institution's policies and the regulatory agencies' standards. A nutrition care plan should[21]

- Be customized for each individual
- Take into account the individual's wishes and preferences
- Include input from the interprofessional team
- Outline several interventions to meet the individual's goals
- Define goal completion date and review schedule
- Be outlined in the medical record

Routine monitoring and adjustment of care plan must take place with changes in medical conditions and when progress toward meeting the patient's goals is not being obtained.

PRACTICE POINTS

Members of the interprofessional team must collaborate to determine the best course of action for each individual patient. Some key points to consider when caring for individuals at risk for or with a PI who are at risk for or malnourished include the following[4,21,47]:

- Implement the use if a validated nutrition screening process to define the nutritional status of individuals with a PI or at risk for developing a PI.
- Individuals screened at risk for malnutrition must be referred to the RDN for the completion of a comprehensive nutrition assessment.
- A patient-centered care plan should be developed for each individual with input from the interprofessional team.
- Educate individuals on the importance of consuming a nutrient dense diet.
- Encourage individuals to consume enriched foods, high-calorie/high-protein ONS, between meals as needed to meet their nutritional needs.
- For individuals with PIs who are at risk for malnutrition or malnourished, as appropriate, recommend the use of ONS enriched with arginine, zinc, and antioxidant to help meet nutritional requirements.
- For individuals who are not able to consume adequate amount of nutrients via PO route, discuss nutrition support (EN and PN).

DISCLOSURE

The author has nothing to disclose.

REFERENCES

1. Edsberg LE, Black JM, Goldberg M, et al. Revised national pressure ulcer advisory panel pressure injury staging system. J Wound Ostomy Continence Nurs 2016;43(6):1–13.
2. VanGilder C, Lachenbruch C, Algrim-Boyle C, et al. The International Pressure Ulcer Prevalence Survey: 2006–2015: a 10-year pressure injury prevalence and demographic trend analysis by care setting. J Wound Ostomy Continence Nurs 2017;44(1):20–8. Available at: https://www.ncbi.nlm.nih.gov/pubmed/27977509. Accessed December 8, 2019.
3. Padula W, Delarmente B. The national cost of hospital-acquired pressure injuries in the United States. Int Wound J 2019;16(10).
4. Haesler E, editor, European Pressure Ulcer Advisory Panel, National Pressure Injury Advisory Panel and Pan Pacific Pressure Injury Alliance. Prevention and treatment of pressure ulcers/injuries: clinical Practice guideline. The international guideline. EPUAP/NPIAP/PPPIA. 2019.

5. Cederholm T, Barazzoni R, Austin P, et al. ESPEN guidelines on definitions and terminology of clinical nutrition. Clin Nutr 2017;36:49–64. Available at: https://www.espen.org/files/ESPEN-guidelines-on-definitions-and-terminology-of-clinical-nutrition.pdf. Accessed December 22, 2019.

6. World Health Organization, Bristol UK. Global Nutrition Report: shining a light to spur action on nutrition. 2018. Available at: file:///Users/nancymunoz/Downloads/2018_Global_Nutrition_Report.pdf. Accessed December 22, 2019.

7. Steiber A, Hegazi R, Herrera M, et al. Spotlight on global malnutrition: a continuing challenge in the 21st century. J Acad Nutr Diet 2015;15(8):1335–41.

8. Sauer AC, Goates S, Malone A, et al. Prevalence of malnutrition risk and the impact of nutrition risk on hospital outcomes: results form nutritionDay in the US. JPEN. 2019. Available at: https://onlinelibrary.wiley.com/doi/full/10.1002/jpen.1499. Accessed December 22, 2019.

9. Goates S, Du K, Braunschweig C, et al. Economic burden of disease-associated malnutrition at the state level. PLOS One 2016;11(9):e0161833. Available at: https://onlinelibrary.wiley.com/doi/full/10.1002/jpen.1499. Accessed Dececmber 22, 2019.

10. Iizaka S, Okuwa M, Sugama J, et al. The impact of malnutrition and nutrition-related factors on the development and severity of pressure ulcers in older patients receiving home care. Clin Nutr 2010;29(1):47–53.

11. Ek AC, Unosson M, Larsson J, et al. The development and healing of pressure sores related to the nutritional state. Clin Nutr 1991;10(5):245–50.

12. Saghaleini SH, Dehghan K, Shadvar K, et al. Pressure ulcer and nutrition. Indian J Crit Care Med 2018;22(4):283–9. Available at: https://www.ncbi.nlm.nih.gov/pmc/articles/PMC5930532/. Accessed Dececmber 22, 2019.

13. Center for Disease Control and Prevention. Adult obesity facts. 2018. Available at: https://www.cdc.gov/obesity/data/adult.html. Accessed December 22,2019.

14. Greco JA 3rd, Castaldo ET, Nanney LB, et al. The effect of weight loss surgery and body mass index on wound complications after abdominal contouring operations. Ann Plast Surg 2008;61:235–42.

15. Vikstedt T, Suominen MH, Joki A, et al. Nutritional status, energy, protein, and micronutrient intake of older service house residents. J Am Med Dir Assoc 2011; 12(6):302–7.

16. Barchitta M, Maugeri A, Favara G, et al. Nutrition and wound healing: an overview focusing on the beneficial effects of curcumin. Int J Mol Sci 2019;20(5):1119.

17. Molnar JA, Underdown MJ, Clark WA. Nutrition and chronic wounds. Adv Wound Care (New Rochelle) 2014;3(11):663–81.

18. Quain AM, Khardori NM. Nutrition in wound care management: a comprehensive overview. Wounds 2015;27(12):327.

19. Iizaka S, Kaitani T, Nakagami G, et al. Clinical validity of the estimated energy requirement and the average protein requirement for nutritional status change and wound healing in older patients with pressure ulcers: a multicenter prospective cohort study. Geriatr Gerontol Int 2014;15(11):1201–9.

20. Breslow RA, Hallfrisch J, Guy DG, et al. The importance of dietary protein in healing pressure ulcers. J Am Geriatr Soc 1993;41(4):357–62.

21. Academy of Nutrition and Dietetics. Nutrition care manual. Academy of Nutrition and Dietetics. 2019. Available at: http://www.nutritioncaremanual.org/. Accessed December 22, 2019.

22. Elia M, Zellipour L, Stratton RJ. To screen or not to screen for adult malnutrition? Clin Nutr 2005;24(6):867–84.

23. Kondrup J, Rasmussen HH, Hamberg I, et al. Nutritional risk screening (NRS 2002): a new method based on an analysis of controlled clinical trials. Clin Nutr 2003;3:321–36.

24. Neelemant F, Kruizenga HM, de Vet HC, et al. Screening malnutrition in hospital outpatients. Can the SNAQ malnutrition-screening tool also be applied to this population? Clin Nutr 2008;27(3):439–46.

25. Grattagliano I, Marasciulo L, Paci C, et al. The assessment of the nutritional status predicts the long term risk of major events in older individuals. Eur Geriatr Med 2017;8(3):273–4.

26. Hengstermann S, Fischer A, Steinhagen-Thiessen E, et al. Nutrition status and pressure ulcer: what we need for nutrition screening. JPEN J Parenter Enteral Nutr 2007;31(4):288.

27. Langkamp-Henken B, Hudgens J, Stechmiller JK, et al. Mini nutritional assessment and screening scores are associated with nutritional indicators in elderly people with pressure ulcers. J Am Diet Assoc 2005;105(10):1590–6.

28. Poulia KA, Yannakoulia M, Karageorgou D, et al. Evaluation of the efficacy of six nutritional screening tools to predict malnutrition in the elderly. Clin Nutr 2012; 31(3):378–85.

29. Trans Tasman Dietetic Wound Care Group. Evidence based practice guidelines for the nutritional management of adults with pressure injuries. 2011. Available at: www.ttdwcg.org. Accessed December 2019.

30. Tsai AC, Chang TL, Wang YC, et al. Population-specific short-form mini nutritional assessment with body mass index or calf circumference can predict risk of malnutrition in community-living or institutionalized a people in Taiwan. J Am Diet Assoc 2010;110(9):1328–34.

31. Nestle Nutrition Institute. Mini nutritional assessment MNA®. Nestlé. 1994. Available at: https://www.mna-elderly.com/forms/mini/mna_mini_english.pdf. Accessed December 2019.

32. BAPEN. Malnutrition universal screening tool. 2003. Available at: https://www.bapen.org.uk/pdfs/must/must-full.pdf. Accessed December 2019.

33. Kondrup J, Allison SP, Elia M, et al. ESPEN guidelines for nutrition screening 2002. Clin Nutr 2003;22(4):415–21.

34. Dutch Malnutrition Steering Group. SNAQ English. Dutch Malnutrition Steering Group. 2019. Available at: https://www.fightmalnutrition.eu/?s=SNAQ+English. Accessed December 2019.

35. Dutch Malnutrition Steering Group. SNAQ (various languages). Dutch Malnutrition Steering Group. 2019. Available at: https://www.fightmalnutrition.eu/?s=SNAQ. Accessed December 2019.

36. Keller HH, Goy R, Kane SL. Validity and reliability of SCREEN II (Seniors in the Community: risk evaluation for eating and nutrition, version II). Eur J Clin Nutr 2005;59:1149–57.

37. Flintbox. SCREEN©: seniors in the community risk evaluation for eating and nutrition. Wellspring Worldwide, LLC. 2016. Available at: https://www.flintbox.com/public/project/2750. Accessed December 2019.

38. Allen B. Effects of a comprehensive nutritional program on pressure ulcer healing, length of hospital stay, and charges to patients. Clin Nurs Res 2013;22(2):186–205.

39. White J. Consensus Statement: AND and ASPEN: characteristics recommended for the identification and documentation of adult malnutrition (undernutrition). J Acad Nutr Diet 2012;112(5):730–8.

40. Hubbard GP, Elia M, Holdoway A, et al. A systematic review of compliance to oral nutritional supplements. Clin Nutr 2012;31(3):293–312.
41. Hartgrink HH, Wille J, Konig P, et al. Pressure sores and tube feeding in patients with a fracture of the hip: a randomized clinical trial. Clin Nutr 1998;17(6):287–92.
42. Arinzon Z, Peisakh A, Berner YN. Evaluation of the benefits of enteral nutrition in long-term care elderly patients. J Am Med Dir Assoc 2008;9(9):657–62.
43. Bourdel-Marchasson I, Dumas F, Pinganaud G, et al. Audit of percutaneous endoscopic gastrostomy in long-term enteral feeding in a nursing home. Int J Qual Health Care 1997;9(4):297–302.
44. Horn SD, Bender SA, Ferguson ML, et al. The National Pressure Ulcer Long-Term Care Study: pressure ulcer development in long-term care residents. J Am Geriatr Soc 2004;52(3):359–67.
45. Dryden SV, Shoemaker WG, Kim JH. Wound management and nutrition for optimal wound healing. Atlas Oral Maxillofac Surg Clin North Am 2013;21:37–47.
46. Wild T, Rahbamia A, Killner M, et al. Basics in nutrition and wound healing. Nutrition 2010;26(9):862–6.
47. Munoz N, Posthauer ME, Cereda E, et al. Nutrition, Essential for Pressure Injury Prevention and Healing: The 2019 International Guideline Recommendations. Advances in Wound Care 2020.

Heel Pressure Injuries in the Adult Critical Care Population

Barbara Delmore, PhD, RN, CWCN, MAPWCA, IIWCC-NYU[a],*,
Elizabeth A. Ayello, PhD, MS, BSN, ETN, RN, CWON, MAPWCA[b]

KEYWORDS

• Pressure injuries • Heel pressure injuries • Critical care • Prevention • Treatment

KEY POINTS

- Because of comorbid diseases and conditions, patients in critical care settings are more vulnerable to pressure injury occurrence.
- The second most common location for pressure injuries is the heel largely because of its structural anatomy and limited blood supply.
- Prevention strategies are the hallmark for avoiding heel pressure injury occurrence.
- Risk factor identification can help the clinician determine those patients more susceptible to heel pressure injury occurrence and apply prevention strategies in a timely fashion.

INTRODUCTION

Knowledge regarding the causes of pressure injuries has advanced over the years, yet pressure injuries are still a pervasive problem. It is understood that there are a multitude of intrinsic and extrinsic risk factors responsible for their cause, but the knowledge needs to be further advanced particularly in vulnerable patient populations, such as patients in the critical care setting.[1–4] Patients in the critical care setting have a multitude of diseases and conditions that contribute to their illness in addition to the risk factors inherent in a critical care setting, such as multiple medications, prolonged ventilation, immobilization, and extended length of stay. The Society for Critical Medicine has listed diagnoses such as respiratory disorders, cardiovascular procedures, septicemia, and severe sepsis as among the top diagnoses in US critically ill patients.[5]

[a] Department of Plastic Surgery, Center for Innovations in the Advancement of Care (CIAC), Hansjörg Wyss, NYU Langone Health, 545 1st Avenue, Greenberg Hall, SC1-160, New York, NY 10016, USA; [b] Advances in Skin & Wound Care, WCET® Journal, Excelsior College, School of Nursing, Hartford Institute for Geriatric Nursing, Ayello, Harris & Associates, Inc, New York, NY, USA
* Corresponding author.
E-mail address: barbara.delmore@nyulangone.org

Crit Care Nurs Clin N Am 32 (2020) 589–599
https://doi.org/10.1016/j.cnc.2020.08.008
0899-5885/20/© 2020 Elsevier Inc. All rights reserved.

A pressure injury is defined as localized damage to the skin and underlying soft tissue. It is usually over a bony prominence due to intense pressure, prolonged pressure, and/or pressure with shear. Pressure injuries can also be related to a medical or other device.[4] Heel pressure injuries are particularly worrisome because they are the number 2 most common anatomic site.[6–14] Like all pressure injuries, heel pressure injuries are likely to occur in vulnerable populations, such as in critically ill patients.

The occurrence of a pressure injury can have negative consequences to the patient and the facility. The patient with a pressure injury may encounter pain, poor quality of life, and possibly mortality.[15] A facility that has caused a pressure injury faces lack of reimbursement, penalties, and possible legal consequences.[16,17] The purpose of this article is to discuss the heel anatomy, scope of the problem, risk factors for heel pressure injuries as they apply to the patient in the critical care setting, and the appropriate strategies that can be used to prevent their occurrence.

THE ANATOMY OF THE HEEL

Understanding the heel anatomy helps to appreciate why the heel can be so vulnerable to a pressure injury. The posterior calcaneus bone, also known as the heel bone, has a large width in relation to its covering skin. The covering skin is approximately 3.8 mm with the epidermis only accounting for 0.46 mm.[18] Therefore, it is largely a small piece of subcutaneous tissue, which is thin, highly vascularized, firm, and fibrous over the calcaneus bone. More importantly, this piece of subcutaneous tissue lacks the muscle tissue required for additional cushioning.[19–21] All of this structural anatomy results in a heel that is underprotected by the skin and thus more vulnerable to damage from pressure and shear forces.

The heel's blood supply is limited. Arterial blood supply arises from the plexus that originates at the posterior tibial and peroneal arteries.[22] Unfortunately, like other areas of the foot, there is not an efficient collateral network, which means that the heel pad relies on arterial flow from the posterior tibial artery's collateral branches.[18,23,24] If a critical care patient has any diseases, conditions, receiving medications during their critical care stay, such as vasoconstrictors, or has experienced any situations, such as prolonged heel positioning without relief, the arterial flow can give rise to ischemic changes to the heel's skin surface, such as is seen in a pressure injury.[6,18,20,22]

HEEL PRESSURE INJURIES IN THE CRITICAL CARE SETTING
Scope of the Problem: Prevalence Estimates and Incidence Data

To define the scope of pressure injury, prevalence estimates or incidence data (to determine hospital-acquired pressure injuries) are measurement methods used. Prevalence is defined as the proportion of patients with a pressure injury divided by the number of all patients studied at a specific point in time. Incidence is defined as the number of patients who develop a pressure injury divided by the total number of patients studied over a specific time period.[25] In the critical care setting, prevalence estimates or incidence data are generally higher than in other care units. Prevalence estimates in adult critical units have been reported to be 8.8% to 33.7%[10,26] Incidence data in the adult critical care units have been reported from 6% to 39.3%.[12,27,28] Kayser and colleagues[29] found that an intensive care unit (ICU) stay made it more likely that a patient developed a pressure injury especially a severe one (full-thickness pressure injury). Heel pressure injury occurrence is often included within reported prevalence estimates and incidence data in the critical care setting, but when isolated, heel pressure injury incidence can range from 9.2% to 17%.[30,31]

It is often difficult to compare hospital-acquired prevalence estimates and incidence data because not all pressure injury stage data may be collected and/or reported, varying formulas may be used to calculate the data, and methodology may differ. However, it is recommended that using the European Pressure Ulcer Advisory Panel (EPUAP), National Pressure Injury Advisory Panel (NPIAP), and the Pan Pacific Pressure Injury (PPPIA) prevalence and incidence formulas contained in the 2019 Clinical Practice Guideline would provide consistency of methodology and more accurate comparisons of prevalence and incidence data possible.[25]

Stages of Heel Pressure Injuries

All pressure injury stages can occur on the heel, but VanGilder and colleagues[32] found that deep tissue pressure injuries (DTPI) were the most frequently occurring stage. In fact, DTPIs occurred at a higher percentage on the heel (41%) than compared with the sacrum or the buttocks (19% and 13%, respectively). Other researchers have found similar results.[13,14] DTPIs present as intact, deep purple, or maroon discoloration or as a blood-filled blister. It can also have areas of nonintact skin that is from epidermal separation[33] and can often be mistaken as a stage 2 pressure injury. This wound generally evolves to a stage 3 or 4 or as an unstageable pressure injury.[13,14] However, some DTPIs may present as a partial-thickness wound[13,14] possibly resolving without tissue loss—a mechanism currently not well understood.[33] DTPIs can be difficult to detect in darkly pigmented patients[33] and may be erroneously labeled as a stage 1 pressure injury. Both stage 1 and DTPIs can present as intact skin, which may serve as the source of confusion; however, the DTPI colors are frequently very deep (maroon, purplish) (**Fig. 1**) and vibrant in presentation and often evolve to an ulceration.

HEEL PRESSURE INJURY RISK FACTORS

Pressure injury formation can be influenced by various intrinsic and extrinsic factors that relate to diseases, conditions, procedures, and the environment. Examples of typical factors are microclimate, nutrition, perfusion, comorbid conditions, and condition of the soft tissue.[4,6,22] The newly released 2019 EPUAP, NPIAP, PPPIA pressure injury clinical practice guideline[15] has a specific good practice statement (#1.18) about risk factors for individuals in critical care. It states: "Consider the following factors to be population specific pressure injury risk factors for critically ill individuals:

- Duration of critical care unit stay
- Mechanical ventilation
- Use of vasopressors
- Acute Physiology and Chronic Health Evaluation (APACHE II Score)."[34(p55)]

Risk factor identification is important because it alerts the clinician to applying timely prevention strategies and possibly preventing a pressure injury particularly on the heel.[18] It has been postulated that there is no single factor that leads to the occurrence of a pressure injury, but more multiple factors present together.[35] In the critical care setting, typical risk factors associated with pressure injuries are age,[12,35–37] prolonged ICU stay,[12,26,35–38] diabetes,[35,36] mechanical ventilation including prolonged mechanical ventilation,[35,36,39,40] hypotension including prolonged hypotension,[26,35,36,39] cardiovascular disease or event,[36,37,39] intermittent hemodialysis or continuous venovenous hemofiltration therapy,[35] shock states,[40] use of vasopressors,[26,35–37,39,40] reduced turning, positioning efforts or mobility,[12,35,37] and prolonged sedation.[35,40] Risk factors that have been linked to heel pressure injury formation are not so different. The most common risk factors are diabetes[6,22,41–43] and vascular disease.[6,22,41,43,44]

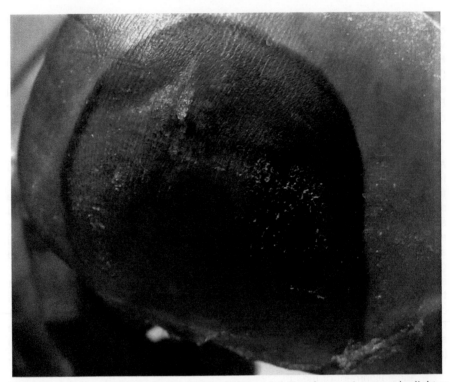

Fig. 1. DTPI of the right heel. Unlike stage 1 pressure injuries that are intact and a lighter red/pink, DTPIs are intact but have a deeper discoloration indicating a deeper level of damage. These full-thickness pressure injuries often evolve to a stage 3 or 4, or an unstageable pressure injury. (© 2019 Delmore).

Other factors include an at-risk pressure injury score,[9,22,43] limited mobility,[9,22] and incontinence.[9] A recent study by Delmore and colleagues[6] on a large population found in addition to diabetes and vascular disease, 5 other significant and independent predictors of heel pressure injuries: perfusion issues, malnutrition, age, mechanical ventilation and surgery. Age is something to carefully consider because the older adult in the critical care setting may be more at risk for heel pressure injury development because the heel's skin and ability to absorb "shock" reduce with age.[45]

HEEL PRESSURE INJURY PREVENTION STRATEGIES

Tayyib and colleagues[12] found that prolonged ICU stays and infrequent repositioning were associated with stages 2 to 4 pressure injury occurrence. This finding is significant because they found that heel pressure injuries were the number 2 location. Their findings for both infrequent positioning as a significant predictor and heel pressure injuries as the second common location may be due to the lack of prevention strategies applied to protect the heel. Prevention strategies have always been touted as a key strategy and remain the hallmark for avoiding heel pressure injury occurrence.[6,11,15,20,46–48]

The recently updated Prevention and Treatment of Pressure Ulcers/Injuries Clinical Practice Guideline[15] has devoted an entire chapter to heel pressure injuries.[49] The Guideline has evidence-based recommendations regarding the prevention and treatment of pressure injuries and is the result of a collaborative effort between the NPIAP, EPUAP, and the PPPIA. It confirms that the heel is the second most common anatomic site and that certain patients are more at high risk for developing a heel pressure injury, including the critical care patient.

This article outlines several recommendations regarding a heel assessment, prevention, and treatment (discussed in this article under section, "Treatment of Heel Pressure Injuries"). The heel assessment points should include the following:

- Assess the vascular/perfusion status of the heel, including skin color, skin temperature, quality of skin, and pulses.
- Check the patient's sensation to the heel.
- Assess patient's risk for developing a pressure injury.
- Assess the patient's clinical condition, medical history, risk factors for developing a heel pressure injury, and history of previous heel pressure injuries.[49]

Prevention strategies recommended include positioning techniques and use of products to offload the heel, thus avoiding pressure injury occurrence. The main point regarding heel pressure injury prevention is that the heels should be free from any surface:

- Elevate the heels using a specifically designed heel suspension device or a pillow/foam cushion.
- Follow the manufacturer's guideline for heel suspension devices.
- When using a heel suspension device or pillow/foam cushion, consider the patient's clinical conditions and preference, such as increased movement from agitation or muscle spasms, skin integrity, including edema, anatomic appearance/alignment of the hip, lower leg, and foot, and the individual's tolerance of the device.
- Positioning aspects in devices should include slight flexion of the knee, high pressure areas, such as under the Achilles tendon, even distribution under the calves, and proper foot alignment avoiding internal/external rotation.
- Remove the heel suspension device periodically (at least twice per day) and more often if edema or fluid shifting is present, to assess the skin's integrity and perfusion status.[49]

It is of note that when using any product or device especially on a critically ill patient, special attention should be used to avoid medical device-related pressure injuries.[50] Because a heel suspension device is recommended as best practice for avoiding a heel pressure injury, it is particularly important that staff ensures that a critically ill patient does not develop a heel, calf, Achilles, or foot pressure injury. It is not uncommon that patients in the critical care setting are experiencing fluid shifting or are edematous. These conditions only make the patient more vulnerable to a heel pressure injury and/or a medical device-related pressure injury.

When viewing the literature, there is much agreement with the recommendations put forth in the 2019 Clinical Practice Guideline. Offloading the heel is considered best practice for avoiding heel pressure injuries. An offloading device that lifts the heel off the bed surface is preferred to pillows because these devices have a better ability to offload the heel, maintain the foot in a neutral position (neither internally or externally rotated; **Fig. 2**), and avoid foot-drop, contracture formation, or additional pressure placed to other parts of the lower leg and foot.[6,19,20,51,52] Prophylactic multilayer foam dressing use in the critical care setting has been reported in the literature as a way to help prevent pressure injuries. However, when using a prophylactic multilayer foam dressing to prevent heel pressure injuries, they are not recommended as the only

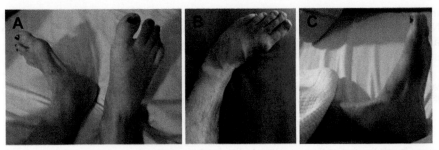

Fig. 2. The left foot in an externally rotated position (*A*), an internally rotated position (*B*), and in the neutral position (*C*). The neutral position is preferred because a foot internally or externally rotated can lead to various issues especially pressure injuries at the lateral malleolus or foot due to improper positioning and increased pressure. (© 2019 Ayello and Delmore).

prevention technique for offloading the heel. Instead, use of multilayer foam dressings should be part of the heel prevention strategies.[6,30,46,49,53–56] In addition, it is recommended that when repositioning a patient, the heels should be repositioned to ensure that they are properly offloaded.[57] The key important components are early identification of patients at risk and early implementation of pressure redistribution and skin protection strategies to help prevent heel pressure injuries in critically ill patients.

HEEL PRESSURE INJURY PREVENTION ENABLER

Research has identified risk factors associated with heel pressure injuries, but the issue is that research findings can take 1 to 2 decades before being enacted in practice.[58] An additional consideration is that clinicians are often inundated with facts and recommendations and experience multiple distractions at the practice setting; this is probably the reason adult learners do well with concepts and learning when presented in a multimodal style.[59] Guides or cues can provide quick information or reinforcement of information and therefore are often needed and appreciated.

With this concept in mind, Delmore and colleagues[6] created an enabler (in a cursory mnemonic form) based on their research findings[6,22] regarding heel pressure injuries and best practice for preventing them. The intent of the enabler is to quickly provide validated heel pressure injury risk factors with recommended prevention strategies that should be applied in a timely fashion to avoid occurrence (**Fig. 3**).

TREATMENT OF HEEL PRESSURE INJURIES

The principles of treating heel pressure injuries include redistribution of pressure by offloading devices, skin protection, and local wound care based on the wound bed preparation paradigm.[60,61]

- *Treat the cause*: Pressure causes pressure injury, so redistribute the pressure. When selecting a heel offloading device, make sure it is the appropriate size especially in persons whose feet are edematous.[60,61]
- *Local wound care*
  - Assess the vascular status of the patient's leg and foot.
  - Do not debride stable heel eschar for patients with untreated peripheral vascular disease; however, "if there is a high suspicion of infection, heel eschars should be debrided to reveal the base of the heel pressure injury."[49(pp152-153),62]

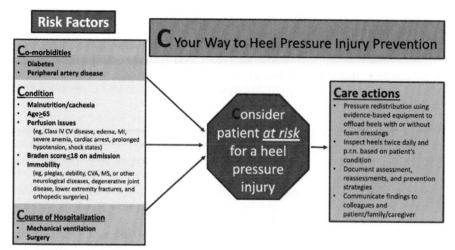

Fig. 3. Heel pressure injury enabler (in a mnemonic format) based on validated risk factors from research conducted by Delmore and colleagues.[6,22] The enabler should be used in conjunction with clinical judgment, individual patient assessment and patient needs and care goals. CV, cardiovascular; CVA, cerebrovascular accident; MI, myocardial infarction; MS, multiple sclerosis. Risk factors represent significant and independent predictors from Delmore et al.[32,35] (© 2019 Delmore, Ayello, & Smart).

SUMMARY

Saving a patient's heel from developing a pressure injury is important. Consider the multiple risk factors that could put a critically ill patient at risk for developing a heel pressure injury. Although a Braden score of 18 or below should trigger the need for prevention strategies, clinicians need to think beyond the validated pressure injury risk assessment tools and consider the individual characteristics of the critically ill patient.

- What medications are they taking?
- Do they affect blood flow to the leg and foot? Is the patient's foot edematous?
- What comorbidities does the patient have: consider their vascular status and if they have diabetes mellitus.

These questions are just some of the considerations in determining if the patient is a risk for a heel pressure injury. Clinicians should not wait to offload the pressure by correctly applying an offloading device, protecting the skin with a multilayer foam dressing, and making sure that the foot is in a neutral position.

DISCLOSURE

The authors have nothing to disclose.

REFERENCES

1. Gould LJ, Bohn G, Bryant R, et al. Pressure Ulcer Summit 2018: an interdisciplinary approach to improve our understanding of the risk of pressure-induced tissue damage. Wound Repair Regen 2019;1–12. https://doi.org/10.1111/wrr. 12730.

2. Coleman S, Nixon J, Keen J, et al. A new pressure ulcer conceptual framework. J Adv Nurs 2014;70(10):2222–34.
3. Coleman S, Gorecki C, Nelson EA, et al. Patient risk factors for pressure ulcer development: systematic review. Int J Nurs Stud 2013;50(7):974–1003.
4. Edsberg LE, Black JM, Goldberg M, et al. Revised National Pressure Ulcer Advisory Panel pressure injury staging system. J Wound Ostomy Continence Nurs 2016;43(6):585–97.
5. Society of Critical Care Medicine. Critical care statistics. The Society of Critical Care Medicine. Available at: http://www.sccm.org/Communications/Critical-Care-Statistics. Accessed January 8, 2020.
6. Delmore B, Ayello EA, Smith D, et al. Refining heel pressure injury risk factors in the hospitalized patient. Adv Skin Wound Care 2019;32(11):512–9.
7. Becker D, Tozo TC, Batista SS, et al. Pressure ulcers in ICU patients: incidence and clinical and epidemiological features: a multicenter study in southern Brazil. Intensive Crit Care Nurs 2017;42:55–61.
8. Lyder CH, Wang Y, Metersky M, et al. Hospital-acquired pressure ulcers: results from the national Medicare patient safety monitoring system study. J Am Geriatr Soc 2012;60(9):1603–8.
9. Muntlin Athlin Å, Engström M, Gunningberg L, et al. Heel pressure ulcer, prevention and predictors during the care delivery chain - when and where to take action? A descriptive and explorative study. Scand J Trauma Resusc Emerg Med 2016;24(1):1–7.
10. VanGilder C, Amlung S, Harrison P, et al. Results of the 2008–2009 International Pressure Ulcer Prevalence™ Survey and a 3-year, acute care, unit-specific analysis. Ostomy Wound Manage 2009;55(11):39–46.
11. Hanna-Bull D. Preventing heel pressure ulcers. J Wound Ostomy Continence Nurs 2016;43(2):129–32.
12. Tayyib N, Coyer F, Lewis P. Saudi Arabian adult intensive care unit pressure ulcer incidence and risk factors: a prospective cohort study. Int Wound J 2016;13(5):912–9.
13. Tescher AN, Thompson SL, McCormack HE, et al. A retrospective, descriptive analysis of hospital-acquired deep tissue injuries. Ostomy Wound Manage 2018;64(11):30–41.
14. Sullivan R. A two-year retrospective review of suspected deep tissue injury evolution in adult acute care patients. Ostomy Wound Manage 2013;59(9):30–9.
15. European Pressure Ulcer Advisory Panel, National Pressure Injury Advisory Panel, Pan Pacific Pressure Injury Alliance. Prevention and treatment of pressure ulcers/injuries: clinical practice guideline. The International Guideline. In: Haesler E, editor. European Pressure Ulcer Advisory Panel, National Pressure Injury Advisory Panel and Pan Pacific Pressure Injury Alliance; 2019.
16. Padula WV, Black JM, Davidson PM, et al. Adverse effects of the Medicare PSI-90 hospital penalty system on revenue-neutral hospital-acquired conditions. J Patient Saf 2018;00(00):1.
17. Fife CE, Yankowsky KW, Ayello EA, et al. Legal issues in the care of pressure ulcer patients: key concepts for healthcare providers–a consensus paper from the International Expert Wound Care Advisory Panel©. Adv Skin Wound Care 2010;23(11):493–507.
18. Salcido R, Lee A, Ahn C. Heel pressure ulcers: purple heel and deep tissue injury. Adv Skin Wound Care 2011;24(8):374–80.
19. Sopher R, Nixon J, McGinnis E, et al. The influence of foot posture, support stiffness, heel pad loading and tissue mechanical properties on biomechanical

factors associated with a risk of heel ulceration. J Mech Behav Biomed Mater 2011;4(4):572–82.

20. Bååth C, Engström M, Gunningberg L, et al. Prevention of heel pressure ulcers among older patients - from ambulance care to hospital discharge: a multi-centre randomized controlled trial. Appl Nurs Res 2016;30:170–5.

21. Guin P, Hudson A, Gallo J. The efficacy of six heel pressure reducing devices. Decubitus 1991;4(3):15–23.

22. Delmore B, Lebovits S, Suggs B, et al. Risk factors associated with heel pressure ulcers in hospitalized patients. J Wound Ostomy Continence Nurs 2015;42(3): 242–8.

23. Faglia E, Caminiti M, Vincenzo C, et al. Heel ulcer and blood flow. Int J Low Extrem Wounds 2013;12(3):226–30.

24. Bosanquet DC, Wright AM, White RD, et al. A review of the surgical management of heel pressure ulcers in the 21st century. Int Wound J 2016;13(1):9–16.

25. European Pressure Ulcer Advisory Panel, National Pressure Injury Advisory Panel, Pan Pacific Pressure Injury Alliance. Measuring pressure injury prevalence and incidence. In: Haesler E, editor. Prevention and Treatment of pressure ulcers/pressure injuries: clinical practice guideline: the international guideline 2019. European Pressure Ulcer Advisory Panel, National Pressure Injury Advisory Panel and Pan Pacific Pressure Injury Alliance; 2019. p. 315–21.

26. El-Marsi J, Zein-El-Dine S, Zein B, et al. Predictors of pressure injuries in a critical care unit in Lebanon: prevalence, characteristics, and associated factors. J Wound Ostomy Continence Nurs 2018;45(2):131–6.

27. Park KH. The effect of a silicone border foam dressing for prevention of pressure ulcers and incontinence-associated dermatitis in intensive care unit patients. J Wound Ostomy Continence Nurs 2014;41(5):424–9.

28. He M, Tang A, Ge X, et al. Pressure ulcers in the intensive care unit: an analysis of skin barrier risk factors. Adv Skin Wound Care 2016;29(11):493–8.

29. Kayser SA, VanGilder CA, Lachenbruch C. Predictors of superficial and severe hospital-acquired pressure injuries: a cross-sectional study using the International Pressure Ulcer Prevalence™ Survey. Int J Nurs Stud 2019;89:46–52.

30. Santamaria N, Gerdtz M, Liu W, et al. Clinical effectiveness of a silicone foam dressing for the prevention of heel pressure ulcers in critically ill patients: Border II Trial. J Wound Care 2015;24(8):340–5.

31. National Pressure Ulcer Advisory Panel. In: Pieper B, editor. Pressure ulcers: prevalence, incidence, and implications for the future. 2nd edition. Washington, DC: National Pressure Ulcer Advisory Panel; 2012.

32. VanGilder C, Macfarlane GD, Harrison P, et al. The demographics of suspected deep tissue injury in the United States: an analysis of the International Pressure Ulcer Prevalence Survey 2006 – 2009. Adv Skin Wound Care 2009;23(6):254–61.

33. National Pressure Injury Advisory Panel. NPIAP pressure injury stages. Available at: https://npiap.com/page/PressureInjuryStages. Accessed January 8, 2020.

34. European Pressure Ulcer Advisory Panel, National Pressure Injury Advisory Panel, Pan Pacific Pressure Injury Alliance. Risk factors and risk assessment. In: Haesler E, editor. Prevention and Treatment of pressure ulcers/pressure injures: clinical practice guideline: the international guideline 2019. European Pressure Ulcer Advisory Panel, National Pressure Injury Advisory Panel and Pan Pacific Pressure Injury Alliance, National Pressure Injury Advisory Panel and Pan Pacific Pressure Injury Alliance; 2019. p. 38–72.

35. Lima Serrano M, González Méndez MI, Carrasco Cebollero FM, et al. Risk factors for pressure ulcer development in intensive care units: a systematic review. Med Intensiva 2017;41(6):339–46.

36. Cox J. Pressure injury risk factors in adult critical care patients: a review of the literature. Ostomy Wound Manage 2017;63(11):30–43.

37. Cox J. Predictors of pressure ulcers in adult critical are patients. Am J Crit Care 2011;20(5):364–75.

38. de Almeida Medeiros AB, da Conceição Dias Fernandes MI, de Sá Tinôco JD, et al. Predictors of pressure ulcer risk in adult intensive care patients: a retrospective case-control study. Intensive Crit Care Nurs 2018;45(4):6–10.

39. Cox J, Roche S. Vasopressors and development of pressure ulcers in adult critical care patients. Am J Crit Care 2015;24(6):501–10.

40. Cox J, Roche S, Murphy V. Pressure injury risk factors in critical care patients: a descriptive analysis. Adv Skin Wound Care 2018;31(7):328–34.

41. Wensley F, Kerry C, Rayman G. Increased risk of hospital-acquired foot ulcers in people with diabetes: large prospective study and implications for practice. BMJ Open Diabetes Res Care 2018;6(1):1–6.

42. Gefen A. The biomechanics of heel ulcers. J Tissue Viability 2010;19(4):124–31.

43. Walsh JS, Plonczynski DJ. Evaluation of a protocol for prevention of facility-acquired heel pressure ulcers. J Wound Ostomy Continence Nurs 2007;34(2):178–83.

44. Meaume S, Faucher N. Heel pressure ulcers on the increase? Epidemiological change or ineffective prevention strategies? J Tissue Viability 2007;17(1):30–3.

45. Cichowitz A, Pan WR, Ashton M. The heel: anatomy, blood supply, and the pathophysiology of pressure ulcers. Ann Plast Surg 2009;62(4):423–9.

46. Schmitt S, Andries MK, Ashmore PM, et al. WOCN society position paper: avoidable versus unavoidable pressure ulcers/injuries. J Wound Ostomy Continence Nurs 2017;44(5):458–68.

47. Ratliff CR, Droste LR, Bonham P, et al. WOCN 2016 guideline for prevention and management of pressure injuries (ulcers): an executive summary. J Wound Ostomy Continence Nurs 2017;44(3):241–6.

48. Haesler E, Rayner R, Carville K. Pan Pacific Clinical Practice Guideline for the prevention and management of pressure injury. Wound Pract Res 2012;20(1):6–20.

49. European Pressure Ulcer Advisory Panel, National Pressure Injury Advisory Panel, Pan Pacific Pressure Injury Alliance. Heel pressure injuries. In: Haesler E, editor. Prevention and Treatment of pressure ulcers/pressure injuires: clinical practice guideline: the international guideline 2019. European Pressure Ulcer Advisory Panel, National Pressure Injury Advisory Panel and Pan Pacific Pressure Injury Alliance; 2019. p. 145–54.

50. Delmore BA, Ayello EA. Pressure injuries caused by medical devices and other objects: a clinical update. Am J Nurs 2017;117(12):36–45.

51. Cuddigan JE, Ayello EA, Black J. Saving heels in critically ill patients. World Counc Enteros Ther J 2008;28(2):16–24.

52. Meyers T. Prevention of heel pressure injuries and plantar flexion contractures with use of a heel protector in high-risk neurotrauma, medical, and surgical intensive care units: a randomized controlled trial. J Wound Ostomy Continence Nurs 2017;44(5):429–33.

53. Ramundo J, Pike C, Pittman J. Do prophylactic foam dressings reduce heel pressure injuries? J Wound Ostomy Continence Nurs 2018;45(1):75–82.

54. Rajpaul K, Acton C. Using heel protectors for the prevention of hospital-acquired pressure ulcers. Br J Nurs 2016;25(6):S18–26.
55. Black J, Clark M, Dealey C, et al. Dressings as an adjunct to pressure ulcer prevention: consensus panel recommendations. Int Wound J 2015;12(4):484–8.
56. Clark M, Black J, Alves P, et al. Systematic review of the use of prophylactic dressings in the prevention of pressure ulcers. Int Wound J 2014;11(5):460–71.
57. Levy A, Gefen A. Computer modeling studies to assess whether a prophylactic dressing reduces the risk for deep tissue injury in the heels of supine patients with diabetes. Ostomy Wound Manage 2016;62(4):42 52.
58. Agency for healthcare research and quality. Translating research into practice (TRIP)-II. Fact sheet. AHRQ publ No 01-P017. 2001;March:1-6. Available at: http://www.ahrq.gov/research/trip2fac.htm%5Cnhttp://www.ahrq.gov/research/trip2fac.pdf. Accessed September11, 2020.
59. Sibbald RG, Alavi A, Sibbald M, et al. Effective adult education principles to improve outcomes in patients with chronic wounds. In: Krasner DL, Rodeheaver GT, Sibbald RG, et al, editors. Chronic wound care 5: a clinical source book for healthcare professionals. 5th edition. Malvern (PA): HMP Communications, LLC; 2012. p. 37–54.
60. Sibbald RG, Goodman L, Woo KY, et al. Special considerations in wound bed preparation 2011: an update. Adv Skin Wound Care 2011;24(9):415–36.
61. Sibbald RG, Ovington LG, Ayello EA, et al. Wound bed preparation 2014 update: management of critical colonization with a gentian violet and methylene blue absorbent antibacterial dressing and elevated levels of matrix metalloproteases with an ovine collagen extracellular matrix dressing. Adv Skin Wound Care 2014;27(3 Suppl 1):1–6.
62. European Pressure Ulcer Advisory Panel, National Pressure Injury Advisory Panel, Pan Pacific Pressure Injury Alliance. Repositioning and mobilization. In: Haesler E, editor. Prevention and Treatment of pressure ulcers/injuries: clinical practice guideline: the international guidleline 2019. European Pressure Ulcer Advisory Panel, National Pressure Injury Advisory Panel and Pan Pacific Pressure Injury Alliance; 2019. p. 115–44.

Pressure Injury Prevention Considerations for Older Adults

Linda Cowan, PhD, APRN, FNP-BC, CWS[a],*, Vianna Broderick, MD[a],
Jenny G. Alderden, PhD, APRN, CCRN, CCNS[b]

KEYWORDS

• Aging • Older • Adult • Pressure • Ulcer • Injury • Risk • Skin

KEY POINTS

• There are significant changes that occur in the human body as it ages.
• Physiologic changes to the skin and supporting structures increase the risk of injury, especially because of mechanical forces of pressure and shearing.
• Multiple factors should be considered in older adults to reduce the risk of pressure injury.

INTRODUCTION

As the older adult population continues to rise, an estimated 20% of all Americans will be older than the age of 65 by 2030. Those older than the age of 85 will likely double from 4.7 million in 2003 to 9.6 million in 2030.[1] Primary aging consists of decreased bone mineral density, decreased muscle mass, abdominal fat accumulation, progressive organ dysfunction, and immunity decline.[2] Secondary aging consists of an accelerated decline because of comorbidities, such as diabetes and hypertension, and lifestyle factors, such as sun exposure and tobacco use.[2] There are many biologic and cellular mechanisms contributing to aging, such as oxidative stress, DNA damage, excess cellular waste, and decreased postmitotic cells and telomeres.[2] As skin ages it becomes uneven in color, thinner, roughened, and wrinkled, possibly leading to impaired wound healing in older adults.[3] With the aging population, the incidence of dermatologic conditions has increased among older adults, leading to more than 27 million annual visits to dermatology clinics.[1]

[a] James A. Haley Veterans Hospital and Clinics, 13000 Bruce B. Downs Boulevard, Tampa, FL 33612-4745, USA; [b] University of Utah College of Nursing, 10 South 2000 East, Salt Lake City, UT 84112, USA
* Corresponding author.
E-mail address: linda.cowan@va.gov

Crit Care Nurs Clin N Am 32 (2020) 601–609
https://doi.org/10.1016/j.cnc.2020.08.009
0899-5885/20/Published by Elsevier Inc.
ccnursing.theclinics.com

Skin is the largest organ of the body, and the only organ system exposed to the direct environment.[3] Aging affects all organ systems but particularly transforms skin appearance via intrinsic and extrinsic factors.[3] Chronologic (intrinsic) aging leads to decreased keratinocyte proliferation and increased water loss, which may impact tissue repair processes.[4] Keratinocytes make up 95% of the skin epidermis layer consisting of stratified and cornified epithelium, forming a barrier, secreting cytokines, and growth factors to maximize skin protection.[4] Melanocytes are the second most common cells in the epidermis impacting skin and hair color. The density of melanocytes decreases with age and contributes to the pallor of older skin and the depigmentation of hair.[4]

The dermis layer provides support beneath the epidermis and is composed of an extracellular matrix with fibroblasts secreting the most abundant protein in human skin: type I collagen.[3] During aging, the type I collagen turnover rate decreases (leading to cross-links) and prevents collagen fragment removal over time.[3] This results in mechanical tension reduction and fibroblast collapse, presenting as thin, fragile, collagen-deficient skin observed in older adults.[3] Aging tends to alter the normal skin pH (typically between 4.5 and 7, slightly acidic to neutral), thereby altering stratum corneum function, reducing lipid processing enzyme action, and diminishing natural skin moisturizers.[5] A study using CBA mice skin samples genetically similar to humans depicted that older mice had epidermal thickness atrophy and fewer pilosebaceous units than younger mice.[6]

Extrinsic aging of the skin is affected by exposure to the environment (eg, sun/ultraviolet exposure, air particulate exposure, chemical exposure). As aging occurs and melanocytes decrease, the skin is more susceptible to sun damage via solar ultraviolet irradiation also known as photoaging.[4,6] Simultaneously, sun damage via solar ultraviolet irradiation (also known as photoaging) further deleteriously affects aging skin.[3] Up to 40% of skin changes in aging are from nongenetic factors. Studies have highlighted nongenetic factors by comparing twins to demonstrate risk factors, such as smoking and history of skin cancer. Overall, skin aging is multifactorial and increases the potential for tissue damage and poor wound healing.[7]

PRESSURE INJURY DEFINITION AND STAGING

Pressure injuries (PrI; formerly known as pressure ulcers) are the result of tissue damage to the skin and underlying structures caused by mechanical forces of pressure and/or shearing forces.[7,8] According to the European Pressure Ulcer Advisory Panel (EPUAP) and the 2019 International Guideline: Prevention and Treatment of Pressure Ulcers/Injuries, stage 1 PrI are typically areas of nonblanchable redness over a bony prominence involving only the epidermal layers of skin (and are potentially reversible). Stage 2 involves epidermal and dermal layers of skin and may present as a clear fluid-filled blister or partial-thickness tissue loss. Stage 3 progresses to full-thickness ulcers involving epidermal, dermal, and subcutaneous tissues, but not fascia, muscle, tendon, cartilage, ligament, or bone (these structures are not visible or palpable in the wound). Stage 4 PrI are full-thickness wounds involving deep tissue structures (muscle, tendon, ligament, bone, and/or cartilage are visible or palpable in the wound). Unstageable PrIs typically present as full-thickness wounds, but where the tissue damage depth cannot be distinguished between stages 3 and 4 because of nonviable or obscuring tissue covering all or part of the wound.

Deep tissue pressure injury (DTPI) is another classification of PrI typically presenting as deep purple discoloration of the skin (or in the wound bed) and/or palpable tissue changes that may or may not eventually evolve to a full-thickness wound.[8-10]

Stage 1 and DTPI PrI may be more difficult to detect in darker pigmented skin given they may appear like bruising or include a blood-filled blister.[8–10] Per the EPUAP Prevention and Treatment of Pressure Ulcers/Injuries 2019 Guidelines, DTPI results from "intense and/or prolonged pressure and shear forces at the bone-muscle interface." PrI to the deep tissues may evolve over several days, where they become covered by thin eschar, or can evolve rapidly and expose deep tissue structures, such as muscle, tendon, or bone (stage 3 or 4 PrI) even with optimal treatment or they may resolve without tissue loss.[8–10] These DTPIs may occur most commonly over the bony prominences of the sacrum, buttocks, and heels, and "pain and temperature change often precede skin color changes."[8–10] The EPUAP cautions, "Do not use DTPI to describe vascular, traumatic, neuropathic, or dermatologic conditions."[8–10]

PATHOPHYSIOLOGY OF PRESSURE INJURY

Many pressure ulcer development theoretic models are based on three or four main interactive components. Defloor's Conceptual Model of Pressure Ulcer Development[11,12] appropriately describes them as:

- Compressive forces: mechanical loads exerting pressure forces on tissue compressed between a bony prominence and another surface, such as a bed or chair.
- Shearing forces: sliding, friction, or rubbing forces exerted on epidermal, dermal, and subcutaneous tissue when a human body moves along a surface, such as sliding up in bed or when transferring to a chair.
- Tissue tolerance for pressure: the ability of internal factors (eg, age, body build, nutrition, hydration, disease burden) to tolerate or withstand external factors (eg, mechanical loads, shear, moisture, environmental assault).
- Tissue tolerance for oxygen: the ability of tissues over bony prominences to respond to internal factors, such as low arterial pressure, poor oxygenation/perfusion, and reperfusion ischemia.

The capability of all four factors to interact with each other influences the level of risk for PrI.[11–14] For instance, if tissue tolerance is high, tissue damage may only occur with longer durations of sustained pressures (eg, over 4 hours), but if tissue tolerance is low, a much shorter duration of pressure may result in tissue damage.[12,14] Gefen[17] suggests PrI may develop in vulnerable body tissue in persons at high risk experiencing sustained mechanical forces for less than 1 hour.

Common PrI risk factors reported in the scientific literature often include but are not limited to advanced age, immobility, urinary and fecal incontinence, nutritional compromise, friction and shear, poor perfusion, sepsis, or comorbid conditions.[11–19] Advanced age is an established risk factor for the development of PrI.[11,13,15,17]

The associated physiologic changes in the human body caused by the aging process increase the risk of injury related to tolerance of mechanical pressure, shearing, and friction forces. Nevertheless, many of the risk factors associated with PrI and DTPI development in older adults are potentially modifiable, such as malnutrition, dehydration, anemia, medication side effects, infection, and urinary and bowel incontinence.[11,13,15,17]

PrI prevention in older adults should address physiologic changes of aging and significant comorbid conditions, adapting interventions aimed at reducing risk related to each specific factor.[15,17] For example, skin integrity in older adults is influenced by internal mechanisms of tissue tolerance and cellular function, interacting with external stressors/forces. Preventive interventions would revolve around minimizing exposure to these external stressors/forces and maximizing cofactors, enhancing the skin's protective function (eg, barrier creams, proactive incontinence care). Appropriate management of comorbid conditions optimizes cellular function in the older adult, and further enhances the skin and underlying tissue's protective function and tolerance to external forces.[19]

DISCUSSION

Table 1 reviews examples of specific aging factors and potential interventions aimed at reducing PrI risk suggested by the scientific literature. This type of table may be a useful format for health care providers of older adults as a quick reference but is by no means comprehensive of every PrI risk factor.

In summary, because of the strong association of older age with PrI risk, and because of the physiologic changes related to aging, all older patients should be considered at risk of PrI. Thoughtful consideration of strategies addressing intrinsic and extrinsic risk factors of PrI risk in older adults include:

- Perform PrI risk assessment to determine level of risk. Using a valid and reliable risk assessment tool for the population of interest is important.
- Performing routine and regular skin assessments of the older adult. It is recommended a thorough head to toe skin examination (including the head and the feet) be conducted consistently and include, but not be limited to, a visual inspection.
- The darkness of the pigment of the skin warrants consideration with skin assessment in darker skinned persons. Skin changes caused by stage 1 and DTPI may be more difficult to determine in darker skinned individuals.[13,26] Relying on visual cues alone is not recommended when assessing the skin over bony prominences in a darker skinned individual. The use of palpation assessing for temperature changes and tissue quality (eg, firm, boggy) is recommended. The evidence for using devices to assist in the assessment of skin over boney prominences (eg, ultrasound, infrared thermographic imaging, pressure monitoring/pressure mapping, and/or subepidermal moisture sensor devices) is gaining research attention and may provide additional objective measures for determining areas of high pressure and early skin damage in individuals of all skin pigmentation types.[25,27,28]
- Address immobility by changing the position of the whole body regularly (at least every 2 hours or less while awake and probably every 4 hours while sleeping). Immobility/decreased activity has repeatedly emerged as a strong, predictive independent risk factor for PrI development.[29] Research demonstrates turning or repositioning a person with limited mobility every 2 hours or less is a standard of care, but other research suggests turning every 4 hours may be adequate to prevent PrI (especially during sleep at night on a pressure redistributing support surface).[14,30] The use of safe patient handling and mobility equipment, such as overhead lift and floor lift devices, "sit-to-stand" devices, and transfer aids, such as lateral air transfer devices, are standard precautions to use to minimize skin injury in immobile individuals (and protect the caregiver from injury).[24,31]
- Using appropriate support surfaces on beds, chairs, and transport devices/stretchers/wheelchairs (check for bottoming out, consider pressure mapping, provide feedback and education to patient and caregivers, document, follow-up plan).[8]

Table 1
Potential interventions to address aging skin challenges

Aging Changes	Pathophysiology	Increases PrI Risk	Possible Preventive Interventions
Thinning tissues	Loss of subcutaneous fat	Loss of protective padding	Reduce pressure and mechanical forces[15,20] Use pressure redistributing support surfaces for bed and chair[20,21] Add external protection from mechanical forces (eg, protective silicone sacral and/or heel dressings)[22,23] Nutritional management (dietitian consultation, optimize nutrition and hydration, address vitamin or mineral deficiencies)[8,15,20]
Rete ridges flatten	Easier separation of epidermis and dermis	Skin more susceptible to shearing forces When a person slides up in bed instead of completely lifting off the bed surface to move them up, the epidermal layer of skin may remain fixed to the bed while the dermal layer, along with the rest of the body, is moved—resulting in tissue separation/damage and often seen as wound undermining in PrIs	Keep the head of the bed as flat as possible to reduce shearing forces from the patient sliding down in bed when sitting up (caution is warranted with aspiration risk)[8] Avoid sliding the patient up in bed or across surfaces during transfers[8] Use safe patient handling and mobility equipment (eg, overhead ceiling and floor lifts) for patient transfers[24]

(continued on next page)

Table 1
(continued)

Aging Changes	Pathophysiology	Increases PrI Risk	Possible Preventive Interventions
Dryer skin	Decreased sebum production, decreased natural skin moisture, and protective barrier	Skin more susceptible to irritants and loss of skin integrity	Avoid drying out the skin with personal skin care and bath products Avoid potential irritants to the skin (perfumed soaps and laundry detergents) Use daily moisturizer for intact skin, especially after bathing Avoid long nails in caregivers to avoid the risk of abrasion
Incontinence (urinary and/or fecal)	Reduced muscle tone of urinary and anal sphincters (may be caused by aging and/or surgical history or comorbid conditions)	Sustained moisture on skin and exposure to effluent acid and enzymes may break down the natural skin barrier, resulting in microclimate changes and inflammation	Address incontinence management (reduce severity of incontinence if possible) Minimize time exposure of skin to urine and feces Consider management devices that prevent contact of effluent with skin, if appropriate Protect skin with barrier creams if exposure to excessive moisture is likely
Heels of feet more susceptible to PrI	Decreased fat tissue and muscle mass (only one layer of panniculus carnosus muscle) in posterior heel combined with small surface area of heel; heel tissues are stiffer and less elastic than in other areas of the foot and body	Pressure exerted directly on calcaneus bone when person is laying down or feet are resting on a footstool or footrests of wheelchair; stiffer soft tissue is less capable of deforming and tolerating strain from pressure	Continue to float heels while patient is in bed or on stretcher and give special attention to heels in wheelchairs or on footstools[25]

Data from Refs.[8,15,20–25]

- Obtain comprehensive nutritional evaluation (including assessment of caregiver's understanding of nutritional needs) and maintain adequate nutrition and hydration.[8,32]
- Optimize hydration, internal and external. Hydrated cells perform better, including the transport of nutrients and waste products across cell membranes. Internal hydration is addressed by adequate fluid intake. External hydration of the skin is also important. This may be addressed by applying gentle moisturizers immediately after bathing and avoiding drying soaps and alcohol-based skin products, if possible.
- Avoid exposure to environmental irritants, including ultraviolet rays; air pollutants, such as tobacco smoke; and caustic chemicals (including urine and stool). Be aware that aging skin may become increasingly sensitive to common substances, such as nickel (found in some jewelry or metallic objects), lanolin (found in many moisturizing creams and lotions or ointments), and neomycin (found in many over-the-counter antibacterial products). Avoid perfumed lotions and check for sensitivity before ordering/using any prescribed ointments/lotions.
- Document, document, document! The critical influence of accurate documentation related to patient assessment, PrI risk factors, skin assessment, interventions implemented, education, and follow-up on patient wellness cannot be underestimated. Studies indicate a need for consistency across disciplines for all PrI-related documentation and further action to improve this important component of health care is warranted.[33]

PrI prevention is an essential component of high-quality health care, particularly among older patients. The development of an age-informed plan of care, including the interventions described previously, is a necessary step toward reducing the incidence of PrI in older people.

DISCLOSURE

The authors have nothing to disclose.

REFERENCES

1. Linos E, Chren M, Covinsky K. Geriatric dermatology—a framework for caring for older patients with skin disease. JAMA Dermatol 2018;154(7):757–8.
2. Fontana L, Klein S. Aging, adiposity, and calorie restriction. JAMA 2007;297(9):986–94.
3. Fisher GJ, Varani J, Voorhees JJ. Looking older: fibroblast collapse and therapeutic implications. Arch Dermatol 2008;144(5):666–72.
4. Yaar M, Gilchrest BA. Ageing and photoageing of keratinocytes and melanocytes. Clin Exp Dermatol 2001;26(7):583–91. Review.
5. Choi EH. Gender, age, and ethnicity as factors that can influence skin pH. In: Surber C, Abels C, Maibach H, editors. pH of the skin: issues and challenges, vol. 54. Basel (Switzerland): Karger; 2018. p. 48–53. Curr Probl Dermatol.
6. Bhattacharyya TK, Thomas JR. Histomorphologic changes in aging skin: observations in the CBA mouse model. Arch Facial Plast Surg 2004;6(1):21–5.
7. Martires KJ, Fu P, Polster AM, et al. Factors that affect skin aging: a cohort-based survey on twins. Arch Dermatol 2009;145(12):1375–9.
8. Pieper B, editor. Pressure ulcers: prevalence, incidence and implications for the future. Washington, DC: National Pressure Ulcer Advisory Panel; 2012.

9. European Pressure Ulcer Advisory Panel, National Pressure Injury Advisory Panel and Pan Pacific Pressure Injury Alliance. In: Haesler E, editor. Prevention and treatment of pressure ulcers/injuries: quick reference guide. The European Pressure Ulcer Advisory Panel: EPUAP/NPIAP/PPPIA; 2019.

10. Edsberg LE, Black JM, Goldberg M, et al. Revised National Pressure Ulcer Advisory Panel pressure injury staging system: revised pressure injury staging system. J Wound Ostomy Continence Nurs 2016;43(6):585–97.

11. National Pressure Ulcer Advisory Panel (NPUAP). NPUAP pressure ulcer stages/categories. Available at: http://www.npuap.org/resources/educational-and-clinical-resources/npuap-pressure-ulcerstagescategories/. Accessed January 27, 2016.

12. Ahn H, Cowan LJ, Lyon D, et al. Risk factors for pressure ulcers including suspected deep tissue injury (sDTI) in nursing home facility residents: analysis of national minimum data set 3.0. Adv Skin Wound Care 2016;29(4):178–90.

13. Defloor T. The risk of pressure sores: a conceptual scheme. J Clin Nurs 1999;8:206–16.

14. Fogerty MD, Abumrad NN, Nanney L, et al. Risk factors for pressure ulcers in acute care hospitals. Wound Repair Regen 2008;16(1):11–8.

15. Gefen A. How much time does it take to get a pressure ulcer? Integrated evidence from human, animal, and in vitro studies. Ostomy Wound Manage 2008;54(10):26–35.

16. Stechmiller JK, Cowan L, Whitney JD, et al. Guidelines for the prevention of pressure ulcers. Wound Repair Regen 2008;16(2):151–68.

17. Komici K, Vitale DF, Leosco D, et al. Pressure injuries in elderly with acute myocardial infarction. Clin Interv Aging 2017;12:1495–501.

18. Lyder CH. Pressure ulcer prevention and management. JAMA 2003;289(2):223–6.

19. Thiyagarajan C, Silver JR. Aetiology of pressure sores in patients with spinal cord injury. Br Med J (Clin Res Ed) 1984;289(6457):1487–90.

20. Jaul E, Barron J, Rosenzweig JP, et al. An overview of co-morbidities and the development of pressure ulcers among older adults. BMC Geriatr 2018;18:305–16.

21. Bolton LL, Girolami S, Corbett L, et al. The Association for the Advancement of Wound Care (AAWC) venous and pressure ulcer guidelines. Ostomy Wound Manage 2014;60(11):24–66.

22. Qaseem A, Mir TP, Starkey M, et al. Risk assessment and prevention of pressure ulcers: a clinical practice guideline from the American College of Physicians. Ann Intern Med 2015;162(5):359–69.

23. Santamaria N, Gerdtz M, Kapp S, et al. A randomised controlled trial of the clinical effectiveness of multi-layer silicone foam dressings for the prevention of pressure injuries in high-risk aged care residents: the Border III Trial. Int Wound J 2018;15(3):482–90.

24. Santamaria N, Gerdtz M, Sage S, et al. A randomised controlled trial of the effectiveness of soft silicone multi-layered foam dressings in the prevention of sacral and heel pressure ulcers in trauma and critically ill patients: the border trial. Int Wound J 2015;12(3):302–8.

25. Oliveira AL, Moore Z, ÓConnor T, et al. Accuracy of ultrasound, thermography and subepidermal moisture in predicting pressure ulcers: a systematic review. J Wound Care 2017;26(5):199–215.

26. American Nurses Association. Safe patient handling & mobility: understanding the benefits of a comprehensive SPHM program. 2015. Available at: https://www.

nursingworld.org/~498de8/globalassets/practiceandpolicy/work-environment/
health–safety/ana-sphmcover__finalapproved.pdf. Accessed January 29, 2016.

27. Cowan L, Mc-Coy-Jones S, Clements C. Clinical look at pressure injuries in darkly pigmented skin. VA Pressure Injury Prevention Field Advisory Group Educational Live Webinar for Clinicians. May 21, 2019.

28. Bates-Jensen BM, McCreath HE, Nakagami G, et al. Subepidermal moisture detection of heel pressure injury: the pressure ulcer detection study outcomes. Int Wound J 2018;15(2):297–309.

29. Bergstrom N, Horn SD, Rapp M, et al. Preventing pressure ulcers: a multisite randomized controlled trial in nursing homes. Ont Health Technol Assess Ser 2014; 14(11):1–32.

30. Gunningberg L, Sedin IM, Andersson S, et al. Pressure mapping to prevent pressure ulcers in a hospital setting: a pragmatic randomised controlled trial. Int J Nurs Stud 2017;72:53–9.

31. Coleman S, Gorecki C, Nelson EA, et al. Patient risk factors for pressure ulcer development: systematic review. Int J Nurs Stud 2013;50:974–1003.

32. Bone P, Buchanan T, Gozzard J, et al. Bariatric safe patient handling and mobility guidebook: a resource guide for care of persons of size. St Louis (MO): VHA Center for Engineering & Occupational Safety and Health (CEOSH); 2015.

33. Chavez MA, Duffy A, Rugs D, et al. Pressure injury documentation practices in the department of veteran affairs: a quality improvement project. J Wound Ostomy Continence Nurs 2019;46(1):18–24.

UNITED STATES POSTAL SERVICE ® Statement of Ownership, Management, and Circulation
(All Periodicals Publications Except Requester Publications)

1. Publication Title	2. Publication Number	3. Filing Date
CRITICAL CARE NURSING CLINICS OF NORTH AMERICA	006 - 273	9/18/20

4. Issue Frequency	5. Number of Issues Published Annually	6. Annual Subscription Price
MAR, JUN SEP, DEC	4	$160.00

7. Complete Mailing Address of Known Office of Publication (Not printer) (Street, city, county, state, and ZIP+4®)

ELSEVIER INC.
230 Park Avenue, Suite 800
New York, NY 10169

Contact Person
Malathi Samayan

Telephone (Include area code)
91-44-4299-4507

8. Complete Mailing Address of Headquarters or General Business Office of Publisher (Not printer)

ELSEVIER INC.
230 Park Avenue, Suite 800
New York, NY 10169

9. Full Names and Complete Mailing Addresses of Publisher, Editor, and Managing Editor (Do not leave blank)

Publisher (Name and complete mailing address)

DOLORES MELONI, ELSEVIER INC.
1600 JOHN F KENNEDY BLVD. SUITE 1800
PHILADELPHIA, PA 19103-2899

Editor (Name and complete mailing address)

KERRY HOLLAND, ELSEVIER INC.
1600 JOHN F KENNEDY BLVD. SUITE 1800
PHILADELPHIA, PA 19103-2899

Managing Editor (Name and complete mailing address)

PATRICK MANLEY, ELSEVIER INC.
1600 JOHN F KENNEDY BLVD. SUITE 1800
PHILADELPHIA, PA 19103-2899

10. Owner (Do not leave blank. If the publication is owned by a corporation, give the name and address of the corporation immediately followed by the names and addresses of all stockholders owning or holding 1 percent or more of the total amount of stock. If not owned by a corporation, give the names and addresses of the individual owners. If owned by a partnership or other unincorporated firm, give its name and address as well as those of each individual owner. If the publication is published by a nonprofit organization, give its name and address.)

Full Name	Complete Mailing Address
WHOLLY OWNED SUBSIDIARY OF REED/ELSEVIER, US HOLDINGS	1600 JOHN F KENNEDY BLVD. SUITE 1800 PHILADELPHIA, PA 19103-2899

11. Known Bondholders, Mortgagees, and Other Security Holders Owning or Holding 1 Percent or More of Total Amount of Bonds, Mortgages, or Other Securities. If none, check box ▶ ☐ None

Full Name	Complete Mailing Address
N/A	

12. Tax Status (For completion by nonprofit organizations authorized to mail at nonprofit rates) (Check one)
The purpose, function, and nonprofit status of this organization and the exempt status for federal income tax purposes:
☒ Has Not Changed During Preceding 12 Months
☐ Has Changed During Preceding 12 Months (Publisher must submit explanation of change with this statement)

PS Form 3526, July 2014 [Page 1 of 4 (see instructions page 4)] PSN: 7530-01-000-9931 PRIVACY NOTICE: See our privacy policy on www.usps.com.

---

13. Publication Title	14. Issue Date for Circulation Data Below
CRITICAL CARE NURSING CLINICS OF NORTH AMERICA	JUNE 2020

15. Extent and Nature of Circulation

			Average No. Copies Each Issue During Preceding 12 Months	No. Copies of Single Issue Published Nearest to Filing Date
a. Total Number of Copies (Net press run)			137	112
b. Paid Circulation (By Mail and Outside the Mail)	(1)	Mailed Outside-County Paid Subscriptions Stated on PS Form 3541 (Include paid distribution above nominal rate, advertiser's proof copies, and exchange copies)	78	57
	(2)	Mailed In-County Paid Subscriptions Stated on PS Form 3541 (Include paid distribution above nominal rate, advertiser's proof copies, and exchange copies)	0	0
	(3)	Paid Distribution Outside the Mails Including Sales Through Dealers and Carriers, Street Vendors, Counter Sales, and Other Paid Distribution Outside USPS®	26	25
	(4)	Paid Distribution by Other Classes of Mail Through the USPS (e.g., First-Class Mail®)	0	0
c. Total Paid Distribution (Sum of 15b (1), (2), (3), and (4))		▶	104	82
d. Free or Nominal Rate Distribution (By Mail and Outside the Mail)	(1)	Free or Nominal Rate Outside-County Copies included on PS Form 3541	18	16
	(2)	Free or Nominal Rate In-County Copies Included on PS Form 3541	0	0
	(3)	Free or Nominal Rate Copies Mailed at Other Classes Through the USPS (e.g., First-Class Mail)	0	0
	(4)	Free or Nominal Rate Distribution Outside the Mail (Carriers or other means)	0	0
e. Total Free or Nominal Rate Distribution (Sum of 15d (1), (2), (3) and (4))		▶	18	16
f. Total Distribution (Sum of 15c and 15e)		▶	122	98
g. Copies not Distributed (See Instructions to Publishers #4 (page 83))		▶	15	14
h. Total (Sum of 15f and g)		▶	137	112
i. Percent Paid (15c divided by 15f times 100)		▶	85.24%	83.67%

* If you are claiming electronic copies, go to line 16 on page 3. If you are not claiming electronic copies, skip to line 17 on page 3.

16. Electronic Copy Circulation

	Average No. Copies Each Issue During Preceding 12 Months	No. Copies of Single Issue Published Nearest to Filing Date
a. Paid Electronic Copies	▶	
b. Total Paid Print Copies (Line 15c) + Paid Electronic Copies (Line 16a)	▶	
c. Total Print Distribution (Line 15f) + Paid Electronic Copies (Line 16a)	▶	
d. Percent Paid (Both Print & Electronic Copies) (16b divided by 16c × 100)	▶	

☒ I certify that 50% of all my distributed copies (electronic and print) are paid above a nominal price.

17. Publication of Statement of Ownership

☒ If the publication is a general publication, publication of this statement is required. Will be printed in the DECEMBER 2020 issue of this publication.

☐ Publication not required.

18. Signature and Title of Editor, Publisher, Business Manager, or Owner

Malathi Samayan - Distribution Controller

Malathi Samayan

Date 9/18/20

I certify that all information furnished on this form is true and complete. I understand that anyone who furnishes false or misleading information on this form or who omits material or information requested on the form may be subject to criminal sanctions (including fines and imprisonment) and/or civil sanctions (including civil penalties).

PS Form 3526, July 2014 (Page 3 of 4)

PRIVACY NOTICE: See our privacy policy on www.usps.com

Moving?

Make sure your subscription moves with you!

To notify us of your new address, find your **Clinics Account Number** (located on your mailing label above your name), and contact customer service at:

Email: journalscustomerservice-usa@elsevier.com

800-654-2452 (subscribers in the U.S. & Canada)
314-447-8871 (subscribers outside of the U.S. & Canada)

Fax number: 314-447-8029

Elsevier Health Sciences Division
Subscription Customer Service
3251 Riverport Lane
Maryland Heights, MO 63043

*To ensure uninterrupted delivery of your subscription, please notify us at least 4 weeks in advance of move.

Printed and bound by CPI Group (UK) Ltd, Croydon, CR0 4YY

03/10/2024

01040483-0013